Instant Pot Type-2 Diabetes Cookbook

365 5-Ingredient or Less Instant Pot Recipes for Type-2 Diabetes People, Help You Live Happily and Comfortable, **Lose Weight and Reverse Your Diabetes**

By Linda C. Jenny

Contents

Forward

Have you been diagnosed with Type-2 Diabetes or on the way to it?

Do you want to make easy diabetic-friendly recipes with your Instant Pot in few minutes?

Do you want to reverse your Type-2 Diabetes or live with it comfortable?

If yes for any questions above, then this book is right for you.

Life with diabetes can be tough, and when you get the news you are pre-diabetic, or developed Type-2 diabetes, your whole world can be turned upside down. All of a sudden you need to make big lifestyle changes, adjust and adapt, and even the smallest of things can feel like an enormous challenge.

One of the principal ways Type-2 diabetes can affect your life is your diet. Before you developed diabetes, chances are your diet was not a serious concern. You might have made some effort to eat healthy, or you might have enjoyed your food with no concerns.

When you have Type-2 diabetes, every single bite counts. It can become very challenging to eat well when this happens. Suddenly you can't always eat out, and when you do you have to look for places with nutritional details on the menu. A lot of your favorite treats are completely off limits, and some regular staples are dangerous for your illness. What's more, some people find that their insulin use contributes to weight gain, or their dietary restrictions cause them to lose too much weight.

This book aims to provide you with simple, delicious, easy to cook meals that will be healthy for you to eat every day, as well as healthy snacks for whenever you are feeling hypo; needing sugar quickly. By sticking to five ingredients or less we make sure we always know what we are eating, and by using the Instant Pot we make sure we can cook something delicious every day.

If you live off the recipes in this book, not only will you be able to manage your Type-2 diabetes better, but you might find that some of your symptoms diminish.

Part 1: Why Instant Pot Cooking?

In the world of multi-functional cooking devices, the Instant Pot reigns as king. It is without a doubt consistently the most innovative, developed, complete product you could possibly wish for in your kitchen. The Instant Pot is a combined slow cooker, pressure cooker, frying pan, pot, bread maker, yogurt maker, and general kitchen tool for cooking absolutely everything.

Because diabetes can often make it difficult to eat a healthy, balanced diet, we need ways of making our diet easier to follow. An Instant Pot allows us to cook healthy meals and snacks with the press of a button, and thanks to its eight pre-set settings, you can rest assured knowing that your food will be cooked to perfection.

How To Use it Effectively?.

There is no magic trick to using an Instant Pot. That's the charm of it. Whatever you want to make, it is pretty intuitive to just hit the right button. And the pre-set, named settings make it even easier.

Of course, like with all things, there is a learning curve. That learning curve with the Instant Pot will be covered as you work through this book. We have 150 recipes for you to try out, as well as charts for cooking time. Maybe you don't feel super confident right now, but after cooking a few of these delicious and simple recipes, you will feel better about using the Instant Pot.

Once you have cooked around ten recipes three times each, you will feel more comfortable doing them from memory, or mixing things up a little. By the time you have made your way through the book you should be a diabetic Instant Pot pro; able to craft amazing meals following the recipes or inventing your own as you go along.

Know About The Buttons And Features.

What ARE all these buttons? Glad you asked! The Instant Pot, depending on your model, has three different types of buttons: pre-set buttons, specific item buttons, and adjusting buttons.

1. Pre-Set Buttons.

These buttons are quite simply normal buttons that are calibrated to cook at a certain pressure or temperature for a certain amount of time. The Instant Pot doesn't know what you've put in, that button is just a safe amount of time for cooking that food type.

MANUAL: Cooks at the highest pressure. Press it and use the + and − buttons to choose your cooking time.

SOUP: High pressure for 20-40 minutes.

MEAT: High pressure for 20-45 minutes.

BEAN: High pressure for 25-40 minutes.

POULTRY: High pressure for 5-30 minutes.

SLOW COOK: No-pressure for a slow cook.

MULTIGRAIN: High pressure for 20-40 minutes.

PORRIDGE: High pressure for 15-30 minutes.

STEAM: High pressure continuous heat.

2. Specific Item Buttons.

Not all Instant Pots have these, but some have buttons for specific items, such as for boiling eggs, baking bread, or making yogurt. These programs are so specific that they will not cook anything else properly.

SAUTE: Brown food with the lid off.

WARM: Keeps food warm and ready for the table without overcooking it.

RICE: Only white rice.

EGGS: Only eggs.

BREAD: Bread maker function.

YOGURT: Ferments yogurt.

3. Adjusting Buttons.

You don't even need to touch these as a beginner Instant Pot user; they alter the program you have selected, or allow you to create your own program.

+ AND -: Increase or decrease times, pressure, and temperatures.

PRESSURE: Swap between high and low pressure.

ADJUST: Adjust settings.

TIMER: Select a cooking button and time, then hit this button and decide how many minutes the Instant Pot should wait before beginning.

How to Maintain the Instant Pot?.

Maintaining your Instant Pot is as simple as using it properly, always cleaning it, and inspecting it before use and before storage.

1: Inspecting before use. Before use, make sure it is in good working order. It doesn't matter whether you are using it for the first time, you are using it for the second time today, or you are using it after taking it out of storage. Make sure all the parts are there, that it is clean, and the cord is safe to use.

2: Using properly. Always use according to directions. Never use it without enough liquid, or with too much liquid. Do not use it when dirty, and do not use the wrong setting. When in doubt, select MEAT or BEAN.

3: Cleaning the lining. The inner parts of the Instant Pot, including the pot itself, the lid, and any insertables, can be washed in the sink or the dishwasher. Use hot, soapy water, scrub clean, and dry well before returning to the pot.

4: Cleaning the main body. Electrical components should never be submerged in water or splashed. Instead, use a damp to gently wipe around the edges and inside. Make sure it is off when you do this.

5: Storing. Make sure that it is clean and dry, that all components are with it, and the cord is wrapped and tied protectively before storing.

6: Follow manufacturer's instructions at all times. Needless to say, as there are countless editions of the Instant Pot. Example: If a recipe asks for a cup of water but the minimum is two, add another cup. If you are cleaning it and the manufacturer requests a specific tool be used, use it.

7: Have a warranty. Even if you do everything right, factory faults and damage during transit are definitely a possibility. Make sure you have a manufacturer's or a retailer's warranty, in case anything happens to your Instant Pot.

Very Useful Tips and Warnings.

When using your Instant Pot, bear in mind there are safe things to do and completely unsafe things to do. When used properly, your Instant Pot is one of the safest kitchen devices you can get. When used wrongly, even a kitchen spoon can be dangerous, and so can your Instant Pot. Follow these DOs and DON'Ts to make sure you are using your Instant Pot safely.

DO...

- keep your Instant Pot clean and tidy at all times.

- use the pre-set programs.

- use the right program for the food you are cooking.

- double check it is sealed and pressure is building properly.

DON'T...

- get the main body wet.

- cook with too little fluid.

- release the pressure faster than the recipe specifies.

- try and break the pressure of the lid before it is ready.

- place the pot on the stove.

- leave food on Warm too long.

- expose your Instant Pot to direct heat.

- leave it unobserved as it cooks.

- allow children or vulnerable adults to use it unattended.

Part 2: Essentials About Type-2 Diabetes

Being diagnosed with Type-2 diabetes can be stressful. You have gone from being a perfectly normal person, possibly even healthy in every other aspect, to having to change a lot of your lifestyle and start taking medication.

Knowing is half the battle. So, what do we know about Type-2 diabetes?

How to Identify If You Have Diagnosed with Diabetes?

Although the only way to know for sure if you have diabetes is a diagnosis from a qualified medical professional, there are subtle signs and symptoms that hint you are pre-diabetic, or developing diabetes.

1. Early Warning Signs.

These signs could mean you are pre-diabetic, or very early diabetes. If caught early enough, you could possibly reverse diabetes. It is important to pay attention to your body and be aware of what is going on.

- Dark skin on the neck, armpits, elbows, knuckles, and knees.

- Thirsty, and urinating often. Water feels like it is going through you.

- Fatigued, tired. Even if you are sleeping well, or can't fall asleep.

- Vision goes blurry or you see white lights often.

2. Diabetes Warning Signs.

These signs rarely show up outside of full diabetes. If you experience any of these symptoms, you need to see your doctor ASAP.

- Dry mouth often. A bit of a weird smell on the breath between meals.

- Hungry and thirsty. More than usual, or even insatiable.

- Urine infections. Without any other explanation. Urine might smell sweet.

- Weight loss, even if you are eating well.

- Frequent headaches. Without any other explanation.

3. Critical Warning Signs.

These signs could mean the person suffering them is in a life-or death battle with diabetic ketoacidosis, and needs to be taken to hospital.

- Vomiting and severe dehydration.

- A strong smell on the breath.

- Hyperventilation and a quick heartbeat.

- Confused and disoriented.

- Fainting, or slipping into a coma.

The Symptoms and Bad Influence of Diabetes You Should Know

Although it may feel as though diabetes on its own is bad enough, the effects of being diabetic can carry on beyond just the superficial things you notice at first. Being diabetic means continually trying to balance your blood sugar, and when your blood sugar is too high or too low this affects your whole body.

Cardiovascular Disease.

Your heart and blood vessels are especially vulnerable to blood sugar spikes, and this increases your risk of most cardiovascular problems.

Nerve Damage.

High blood sugar can actually burn or kill the tiny blood vessels that lead to your nerves. This can lead to phantom pain, numbness, digestive problems like nausea or constipation, and even erectile dysfunction.

Kidney Damage.

Because your kidneys do the job of filtering out the excess sugar in your blood, if you have a lot of sugar passing through them you can damage these delicate organs. Severe damage can lead to kidney failure or end-stage kidney disease; which could require dialysis or a transplant.

Hand and Foot Damage.

As your nerves and blood vessels die, sometimes tissue in your hands and feet can develop infections and begin to rot.

Eye Damage.

If the blood vessels and nerves in your eyes are affected, you can experience partial or complete blindness, or develop cataracts or glaucoma.

Skin Infections.

As with hand and foot damage, any cuts to your skin heal badly and rot, causing infections and sores.

Urine Infections.

The sugar in your urine makes you more vulnerable to UTIs.

Alzheimer's Disease.

Sometimes called Type-3 diabetes, Alzheimer's is much more common in people who have diabetes or poor blood sugar control.

Birth Defects and Stillbirth.

Pregnant women with diabetes are more likely to give birth to very large babies, babies with low blood sugar, or have a stillbirth.

Preeclampsia.

Preeclampsia is more common in women with diabetes, and can be life-threatening to both mother and baby.

Differences between Type-1, Type-2, gestational, and pancreatic Diabetes.

Although all forms of diabetes, if unmanaged, will affect your body the same way, not all types are equal. Depending what caused your diabetes, it can be classified into one of four common types. Some types can even be completely reversed if you eat well, take your medications, and follow your doctor's advice.

Type-1.

Type 1 diabetes refers to a whole range of autoimmune conditions, where your body attacks the cells in your pancreas that make insulin. It is normally inherited, you will have it your whole life, and 5-10% of diabetics have this type.

Type-2.

Type-2 diabetes refers to diabetes you develop as a consequence of a combination of genes and poor lifestyle choices. Some people are more vulnerable than others, but generally it can be managed with better lifestyle choices. 90% of diabetics have this type.

Gestational.

During pregnancy the placenta releases hormones, which can affect how you use insulin. Normally your body will produce more insulin and rebalance, but when this doesn't happen you can develop gestational diabetes. 2-4% of pregnant women develop this.

Pancreatic.

When you have pancreatitis, a part of your pancreas can become inflamed or even die. If you have cancer of the pancreas, your pancreas may be removed. If you lose some of your pancreas, you can lose your ability to produce enough insulin.

<u>Another type?</u>

This is not the end of the list. There are more types of diabetes out there. For example, a baby can be born with Neonatal Diabetes, which is different from Type-1 or Type-2. People with MODY diabetes do not need insulin. People on steroids can spontaneously develop diabetes. Make sure you know what type of diabetes you have.

How Can I Prevent Diabetes?

Some forms of diabetes, unfortunately, cannot be prevented. If you have Type-1, juvenile, or pancreatic diabetes, then chances are it was mostly, if not entirely, down to fate.

However, some types of diabetes can be prevented with careful management, and most of the time, the same things that help with one will also help with other types. The most commonly preventable type of diabetes is Type-2. Type-2 diabetes can be avoided by maintaining a healthy weight, exercising 10 minutes a day or 30 minutes twice a week, consuming less sugar, and not drinking too much alcohol.

Another preventable form of diabetes is when people give themselves pancreatitis. If you eat too much fat and develop gallstones, your pancreas can fail. Smoking can also lead to pancreatitis or pancreatic cancer. And alcoholism, or drinking daily for many years, can cause pancreatitis in some people. If you are at risk, avoid alcohol, tobacco, and oily foods.

Finally, it is also important to remember that even if you cannot prevent yourself from developing diabetes or pre-diabetes, you can definitely hinder its progression. You can also stop it from developing into other health conditions or complications. A healthy diet and lifestyle are essential when it comes to controlling diabetes and managing it.

If you are at risk of any other conditions, for example if you have a family history of pancreatic cancer, or if you have suffered a heart attack, make sure to discuss this with your doctor in detail, so they can make sure that you are getting the support you need in order to prevent your diabetes from making your risk of these conditions even worse.

Is it Possible to Cure It with Diet?

It is important to remember at all times that diabetes *cannot* be cured with diet alone. Many health gurus and nutritionists will tell you they can cure your diabetes because they want to sell you a book, or a three-week course. The reality is that there are many factors that come together to cause diabetes, and diet is only one of them.

If you want to reverse your diabetes, first of all you need to know if it is reversible. A simple test is to ask yourself whether you caused your diabetes, or whether it happened on its own. If your diabetes developed due to things beyond your control, you may not be able to reverse it.

A healthy diet can go a long way towards managing your diabetes, but you will need other things as well. Exercise, medication, supplements, or even surgery may be required to make you healthier. Talk to your doctor, or, ideally, a specialist, about what it would take to reverse your type of diabetes.

And bear in mind that just because you are doing all the right things does not mean your diabetes will magically go away. Maybe there were many factors, one of them being genetic, and you cannot get rid of your diabetes. Maybe you can be symptom-free for a long time, but relapse every time you eat high risk foods. Or maybe you can reverse your diabetes, but some of the complications, such as heart or kidney problems, do not go away.

The most important thing to remember is that any improvement, however small, is for the better. Even if you cannot cure your diabetes, just making your everyday life easier and your health a bit better is worth its weight in gold.

Can I Stop Taking My Prescription?

An important factor, when dealing with *any* condition is to follow your doctor's advice.

There are some signs, however, that you might not need a prescription, and if you experience any of these you want to talk to your doctor about reducing, swapping, or stopping your prescription. Just remember not to do anything without proper medical advice.

1. **The effect of the medication is less than you need.** You may need stronger medication.

2. **The effect of the medication is too severe.** You may need less medication.

3. **There are side effects that make using the medication unpleasant, difficult, or impossible.** You may need a completely different medication.

4. **You have been on this medication for the amount of time your doctor, or the package says you need it.** You need a medication review.

5. **You have lost, or gained, a lot of weight.** You may need a new dose, or a different medication.

6. **The cause of the diabetes has gone.** If you had steroid-induced diabetes, pancreatitis leading to diabetes, or gestational diabetes, sometimes it can heal on its own.

Some people decide to stop taking their insulin as a weight loss method. This is incredibly dangerous and should never be done. If you need a certain dose of insulin after a meal, or because your blood sugar is spiking, then you have to take it. Otherwise, you could eventually begin to suffer a number of complications; which could make you seriously ill or even kill you.

For more information about diabetes and weight management, or the problems with not managing your insulin, read sections, "A Healthy Diet Can Help Weight Loss," and "Important Tips and Warnings For Managing Diabetes" later on in this chapter.

Should I Do More Exercise?

The answer to this question is pretty much always "yes." Exercise benefits pretty much everyone, and if you have diabetes you are no exception. Exercising when you are diabetic can help to burn excess blood sugar, which will keep your blood sugar much healthier than if you did not exercise. Exercise can also stabilize your hormones, encouraging your body to produce more insulin, to balance your hunger hormones, and to manage your insulin production better in general.

A caveat: high blood pressure.

If you have high blood pressure you should still exercise, of course, but you need to go about it a little differently to someone who does not have high blood pressure. You want to start very slow and steady, and make sure to monitor your pulse and blood pressure before, during, and after exercise, so you know you're not pushing your heart too hard. Consider starting with something very low intensity, like walking or swimming, to build your strength up.

A huge caveat: if you are hypoglycemic.

Sometimes when we have diabetes we can use too much insulin. Maybe our blood sugar was going down a bit better than usual, or maybe our monitor gave us the wrong reading, or maybe we just injected way too much insulin. You will find yourself crashing, feeling ill and dizzy, and your strength will diminish. In extreme cases you can faint, or even die. If you are hypoglycemic the last thing you need to do is waste your valuable energy on exercise. And if you keep going hypoglycemic it is important not to overexert yourself until your doctor finds out what is causing your hypoglycemia.

Optimism Is Important.

Because many people who develop Type-2 diabetes develop it through a combination of genes, environment, and lifestyle, it is a sort of cruel irony that now they cannot do many of the things they enjoy. If you have Type-2 diabetes, chances are you are a laid back sort of a person who loves good food and drinks casually. **Three things that can make your diabetes worse: too much time resting, foods high in carbohydrates and fat, and alcohol.** It may seem as though it has robbed you of some of the best things in life.

If you have Type-2 diabetes, all hope is not lost. You can easily control your diabetes with medication and lifestyle changes. And by taking your medication and changing your lifestyle, you can actually get your diabetes controlled enough that you can start enjoying your favorite foods, drinks, and pastimes again. So, even if at first you are not able to eat meals out, drink alcohol, or spend all day relaxing on a Sunday, rest assured that after a few weeks of hard work you can begin adding these things back into your life.

You can massively improve your quality of life with a few simple changes. Once your health is under control you can start following the 80/20 rule; eat low carb, low fat meals 80% of the time, then have pizza, or piece of cake, or something equally indulgent, 20% of the time.

If you cannot improve your health enough so that you can eat and drink the things you used to love, start looking for alternatives. Most sodas make sugar free versions that taste almost exactly the same as the original, and there are many cakes, sweets, and preserves made without sugar, specially for diabetics. Look for these items.

A Healthy Diet Can Help Weight Loss.

As we briefly mentioned above, some diabetics engage in the dangerous practice of skipping their insulin so as to lose weight. This works because all that sugar that your insulin helps you burn or store doesn't go into your fat any more. Where does it go?

Well... nowhere.

And that is precisely the problem. All that sugar floating around in your blood is causing damage to your entire body, burning blood vessels and nerves, rotting your organs, feeding the bacteria that cause UTIs, and damaging your brain.

If you want to lose weight, the only way to do it is to reduce the calories in your body. Healthy ways of doing this include exercising to burn of the excess calories, eating fewer calories so we use more of them, or, if your doctor advises, weight loss surgery to make your stomach smaller, so fewer calories fit into your body. All of these methods work, and are much better for you, as they are safe, compatible with your medication, and easy for your doctor to track.

Keep in mind that not all diets are created equal. Even though a person without diabetes can follow an all-carb diet, a junk food diet, or a cake-based diet and lose weight as long as their calories are lower, these diets are a very bad idea for someone with diabetes.

What is more, an unhealthy diet is an unrealistic way of losing weight. If your diet is not something you can safely follow forever, it is not a safe way to lose weight. If you follow a fad diet, or crash your weight, then as soon as you go back to eating normally you will gain it all back, and maybe more. You need to eat healthy to lose weight safely.

The Ideal Nutritional Balance.

What makes a good diet for a diabetic?

No matter what type of diabetes you have and what your medication, exercise, or long term healthcare plans are, your ideal diet is actually going to be quite similar to any other diabetic's diet. Starting with nutritional balance, you need to make sure you are eating the right ratio of fat, protein, and carbohydrate. You also need to make sure you are eating the right types of carbohydrate, as there are vast difference between carbohydrates; healthy and unhealthy varieties.

Your carbohydrate needs are actually no different as a diabetic than they were before diabetes. You still need, at most, 50% of your calories from carbohydrates, which equals 300g. However, if you are used to eating less, try and eat less. Fats are not as harmful as we have been made to believe, and a diet with healthy fats is no problem. Just be careful if your gallbladder is affected, and avoid trans fats. Also remember, protein can be broken down into glucose, so if you eat a meal high in proteins you must check your blood sugar one or two hours after eating.

Finally, you need to consider what micronutrients you are getting and what ones you need. Our micronutrients come in four types: vitamins, minerals, antioxidants, and fiber. Make sure to eat a balanced amount of all the necessary vitamins and minerals. Pay special attention to Vitamin D; it regulates hormones and helps you make insulin, and chromium, which lowers your blood sugar levels.

When it comes to antioxidants, consider a trans resveratrol supplement to help your body heal and reduce inflammation. Another suggestion concerns fiber; make sure to eat the recommended amount, and ideally twice the recommended amount. This slows down digestion; preventing blood sugar spikes and hunger.

Foods That Are Good for Diabetics.

When you have diabetes it can feel as though there is nothing you can eat any more. Rest assured there are plenty of perfectly safe foods if you know where to look. In fact, there are plenty of foods that will improve your symptoms and make your life easier.

- Whole grains.

- Low carb tubers and roots.

- Fresh, frozen, or raw vegetables.

- Fresh fruit with a high fiber content.

- Fresh berries with a low sugar content.

- Non-sweet fruits.

- Sugar-free and calorie-free products.

- Freshly boiled beans. Tinned and refried beans are higher in simple carbs.

- Nuts and seeds: dry roasted or raw; walnuts, almonds, pistachios, peanuts.

- Fresh meat.

- Whole dairy.

- Black coffee.

Foods That Are Bad for Diabetics.

All that said, there is a host of foods you really should not be eating when you are diabetic. Some of these are common knowledge, but there are others which everyone seems to assume are great for diabetics because they are low in carbs, high in protein, or high in fiber, yet they are actually so high on the glycemic index (GI), they are actually dangerous.

- White grains. This includes "whole wheat" and "whole meal." If it is not "wholegrain," it is out.

- Potatoes. Sweet potatoes are often considered safe, but their GI is very high.

- Breakfast cereals.

- Sweet, squishy fruits. Avoid fruits like bananas, mangoes, or melons that are high in sugar and not as high in fiber as other fruits.

- Canned fruits. They are always preserved in syrup or juice.

- Jelly and jam. Choose ones specially formulated for diabetics.

- Breadcrumbs.

- Deep fried foods.

- Gravies and sauces.

- Low fat dairy (sweetened).

- Sugary drinks.

- Beer.

- Fruit juice.

- Smoothies.

- Flavored hot drinks.

Important Tips and Warnings for Managing Diabetes.

Living with diabetes can feel like a bit of a minefield, so here is a list of simple DOs and DON'Ts that will help you work out some of the most common, least talked about, or most dangerous aspects of this condition.

Do's...

- take medications prescribed, in the amounts prescribed.

- test blood sugar regularly and record the results.

- wear a medical bracelet or other item warning you are diabetic.

- use insulin after a meal, an hour or two after eating protein, or when blood sugar tests high.

- carry insulin and a sweet snack, to balance your glucose.

- follow a healthy diet 80% of the time.

- exercise regularly.

- eat a balance of protein, complex carbohydrate, fat, and fiber at every meal for slow and easy digestion.

- have a snack between meals to maintain a steady blood sugar.

- try and lose weight to help reduce the impact of diabetes.

- manage stress, tiredness, and mental health properly – this helps prevent overeating.

- stay hydrated.

Don'ts...

- forget to check blood sugar.

- skip insulin for weight loss – this could seriously hurt or kill – the best way to lose weight is with diet and exercise.

- use insulin if blood sugar is not high enough.

- eat things that will spike blood sugar.

- eat anything from a fast food place – processed food can be so broken down that the carbs release as pure sugar.

- drink smoothies – blending releases the sugar.

- ignore cuts or sores – they could get much worse.

- skip meals, at least have something small.

Part 3: Diabetics Instant Pot Recipes

Why Only 5-Ingredients or Less?

Getting to the 'meat' of the book, you are probably wondering why we are cooking using only five ingredients or less. After all, to most of us that may sound a bit restrictive, right?

Well, in reality, cooking with five ingredients or less has countless benefits.

First, makes sure you know what's in your food. When you use a few, simple ingredients you know what you are eating, offering peace of mind and comfort.

Second, makes it easier to track your food's nutritional values. Whether you are tracking your diet for your doctor or reducing your calories for weight loss, a simple, five-ingredient recipe is easier to keep a record of.

Third, makes it easy to cook. Fewer ingredients means less prep time, which means you can spend more time doing the things that really matter to you.

Fourth, makes it easy to shop. By focusing on five ingredients or less you restrict your shopping list, allowing you to eat healthy on a budget, or with a tight schedule.

Fifth, the food is guaranteed to be delicious. There is a Hare Krishna principle that says when you cook food natural and simple you don't need to taste it as you cook it, and you will know that it is good. When you use only five ingredients, you know how they will work together, making your food delicious.

Finally, food can be adapted to suit any palate. When you have only five ingredients, you are working with a simple blend you can adapt easily. You could not swap the tomato in a curry for anything else without ruining it, but you can easily swap the tomato in a five vegetable stir fry if you do not like tomatoes.

Notes of Cooking Times.

Cooking times for the Instant Pot vary, and it really depends on what you are cooking and how. Lots of variables can affect how we cook and how long it takes to complete a recipe. The times given at the start of the recipes are estimates; help you work out more or less how much time you will need.

The times are divided into prep and cooking. Prep time is the total time it will take to get the meal ready before placing it in the Instant Pot. If the ingredients list "diced chicken," assume it needs to be diced before prep begins.

To get as close to the prep and cook time are appropriate, take into consideration...

1: The prep time is an estimate based on how long, on average, it takes to carry out all the prep tasks. If you need to do more prep, add extra time.

2: If you have any physical condition that stops you from carrying out prep quickly, then you need to add extra time, or to buy some of your ingredients pre-prepared.

3: Cooking times assume you will cut the food into the same, approximate size stated in the recipe; smaller pieces cook faster, thicker pieces cook slower.

4: Cooking time is total cooking time. If you need to pause halfway through to add something, both cooking sessions will be added for total cooking time.

5: When cooking from dry or from frozen, add extra time. Approximately 20% should do.

6: When pre-cooking any ingredients, remove some time, or add them closer to the end. A fully cooked ingredient only needs 1-5 minutes to heat through in the Instant Pot.

Notes of Ingredients.

The ingredients listed in these recipes are all safe for a diabetic diet so long as they are in that recipe. It is important to remember different foods have different qualities, depending on how you cook them and what you serve them with. Some diabetics can have chocolate, for example, but only with nuts to slow down the digestion process.

For this reason, it is very important to follow the recipes closely. Feel free to mix and match spices and herbs, depending on your needs, as these have very little impact. This will give you variety in your flavors without putting your health at risk.

When it comes to fats, carbohydrates, or proteins, make sure any substitute is like for like. For example swapping chicken for tofu, or brown rice noodles for wholegrain wheat noodles. This means you will not be making substitutions based on flavor, but rather based on the impact they will have on your diet.

Each recipe tracks calories, carbohydrate, sugars, GI, and GL of your food; if any recipe does not meet your requirements for the day, consider making a substitution for any of the following:

Low carb alternatives:

- Squash
- Pumpkin
- Konjac
- Cauliflower
- Almond flour

- Coconut flour
- Coconut chips

Low sugar alternatives:

- Stevia
- Sweeteners
- Berries

Low GL alternatives:

- Wild rice
- Pumpernickel
- Oatmeal
- Quinoa
- Couscous
- Pearl barley
- Celeriac
- Swede

Low calorie alternatives:

- Fat free Greek yogurt
- Kale chips
- Tofu
- Berries
- Konjac

High protein alternatives:

- Tofu

- Kidney beans
- Lean chicken
- Lean beef
- Seafood
- Fat free Greek yogurt

Easy Healthy Breakfasts

When you need something good and healthy for breakfast, diabetes can be a real nightmare. Most breakfast foods are white bread, sugary cereals, or even pastries. So what do we do when these foods are not on the menu? We improvise, of course.

SPICY TOFU SCRAMBLE

Prep time: 15 minutes   **Setting:** Steam
Cooking time: 7 minutes   **Serves:** 2
Nutrition per serving:
Calories: Sugar: 2   Protein: 18
Carbs: 7   Fat: 3   GL: 2
Ingredients:
- 1 cup firm silken tofu
- 1tsp cayenne pepper
- 1tsp chili paste
- 1tsp soy sauce
- pinch of salt

Recipe:
1. Spray a heat-proof bowl that fits in your Instant Pot with nonstick spray.
2. Chop the tofu finely.
3. Stir in the remaining ingredients.
4. Pour into the bowl.
5. Place the bowl in your steamer basket.
6. Pour 1 cup of water into your Instant Pot.
7. Lower the basket into your Instant Pot.
8. Seal and cook on low pressure for 7 minutes.
9. Depressurize quickly.
10. Stir well and allow to rest, it will finish cooking in its own heat.

BREAKFAST BEANS

Prep time: 15 minutes
Cooking time: 10 minutes
Nutrition per serving:

Setting: Stew
Serves: 2

| Calories: 300 | Sugar: 4 | Protein: 42 |
| Carbs: 29 | Fat: 7 | GL: 13 |

Ingredients:
- 1lb baked beans
- 1lb chopped mixed lean meats
- 1 cup scrambled eggs
- 1tbsp mixed herbs
- 2 stalks scallions

Recipe:
1. Mix all the ingredients in your Instant Pot.
2. Cook on Stew for 10 minutes.
3. Release the pressure naturally.

CHEESY EGGS

Prep time: 15 minutes
Cooking time: 7 minutes
Nutrition per serving:

Setting: Steam
Serves: 2

| Calories: 100 | Sugar: 0 | Protein: 16 |
| Carbs: 3 | Fat: 8 | GL: 1 |

Ingredients:
- 3 eggs
- 1/4 cup of milk
- 2tbsp grated cheddar
- 1tsp mixed herbs
- pinch of salt

Recipe:
1. Spray a heat-proof bowl that fits in your Instant Pot with nonstick spray.
2. Whisk together the eggs, milk, salt, and herbs. Pour into the bowl.
3. Place the bowl in your steamer basket.

4. Pour 1 cup of water into your Instant Pot. Lower the basket into your Instant Pot.
5. Seal and cook on low pressure for 7 minutes. Depressurize quickly.
6. Add the cheese.
7. Stir well and allow to rest, it will finish cooking in its own heat.

EGGS AND BACON

Prep time: 15 minutes   **Setting:** Steam
Cooking time: 7 minutes   **Serves:** 2
Nutrition per serving:

Calories: 230	Sugar: 0	Protein: 19
Carbs: 3	Fat: 12	GL: 1

Ingredients:
- 3 eggs
- 1/4 cup of milk
- 1/4 cup chopped bacon
- 1tsp smoked paprika
- pinch of salt

Recipe:
1. Spray a heat-proof bowl that fits in your Instant Pot with nonstick spray.
2. Whisk the eggs and slowly add the other ingredients.
3. Pour into the bowl. Place the bowl in your steamer basket.
4. Pour 1 cup of water into your Instant Pot. Lower the basket into your Instant Pot.
5. Seal and cook on low pressure for 7 minutes. Depressurize quickly.
6. Stir well and allow to rest, it will finish cooking in its own heat.

EGGS AND TOMATO

Prep time: 15 minutes   **Setting:** Steam
Cooking time: 7 minutes   **Serves:** 2
Nutrition per serving:

Calories: 110	Sugar: 2	Protein: 16
Carbs: 5	Fat: 8	GL: 2

Ingredients:

- 3 eggs
- 1/4 cup of milk
- 1 cup chopped cherry tomatoes
- 1 tsp mixed herbs
- pinch of salt

Recipe:
1. Spray a heat-proof bowl that fits in your Instant Pot with nonstick spray.
2. Whisk together the eggs, milk, salt, and herbs.
3. Pour into the bowl. Add the tomatoes. Place the bowl in your steamer basket.
4. Pour 1 cup of water into your Instant Pot. Lower the basket into your Instant Pot.
5. Seal and cook on low pressure for 7 minutes. Depressurize quickly.
6. Stir well and allow to rest, it will finish cooking in its own heat.

SAUSAGE BREAKFAST CASSEROLE

Prep time: 15 minutes
Cooking time: 10 minutes
Setting: Stew
Serves: 2
Nutrition per serving:

Calories: 360	Sugar: 2	Protein: 35
Carbs: 10	Fat: 24	GL: 11

Ingredients:
- 1lb cooked chopped sausage
- 1lb chopped bell pepper and onions
- 1 cup low sodium broth
- 1tbsp mixed herbs
- soy sauce

Recipe:
1. Mix all the ingredients in your Instant Pot.
2. Cook on Stew for 10 minutes.
3. Release the pressure naturally.

HAZELNUT CHOCOLATE OATS

Prep time: 10 minutes

Cooking time: 5 minutes

Nutrition per serving:

Setting: Manual

Serves: 2

| Calories: 300 | Sugar: 3 | Protein: 12 |
| Carbs: 25 | Fat: 9 | GL: 17 |

Ingredients:

- 0.5 cup high fiber steel cut oats
- 2 cups milk
- 4tbsp hazelnuts
- 2tbsp powdered sweetener
- 2tbsp very dark chocolate chips

Recipe:

1. Pour the milk into your Instant Pot.
2. Add the oats and sweetener, stir well.
3. Seal and close the vent.
4. Choose Manual and set to cook 5 minutes.
5. Release the pressure naturally.
6. Top with hazelnut and chocolate.

EGGS AND MUSHROOM

Prep time: 15 minutes

Cooking time: 7 minutes

Nutrition per serving:

Setting: Steam

Serves: 2

| Calories: 100 | Sugar: 0 | Protein: 16 |
| Carbs: 4 | Fat: 8 | GL: 1 |

Ingredients:

- 3 eggs
- 1/4 cup of mushroom soup
- 1 cup chopped mixed mushrooms
- 1tsp mixed herbs
- pinch of salt

Recipe:

1. Spray a heat-proof bowl that fits in your Instant Pot with nonstick spray.
2. Whisk together the eggs, soup, salt, and herbs.

3. Pour into the bowl. Add the mushrooms. Place the bowl in your steamer basket.
4. Pour 1 cup of water into your Instant Pot. Lower the basket into your Instant Pot.
5. Seal and cook on low pressure for 7 minutes. Depressurize quickly.
6. Stir well and allow to rest, it will finish cooking in its own heat.

SPANISH EGGS

Prep time: 15 minutes
Cooking time: 7 minutes
Nutrition per serving:

Setting: Steam
Serves: 2

Calories: 125	Sugar: 1	Protein: 16
Carbs: 5	Fat: 8	GL: 1

Ingredients:
- 3 eggs
- 1/4 cup of milk
- 1 cup shredded, fried onion
- 1 tsp smoked paprika
- pinch of salt

Recipe:
1. Spray a heat-proof bowl that fits in your Instant Pot with nonstick spray.
2. Whisk together the eggs, milk, salt, and paprika.
3. Pour into the bowl. Add the onion. Place the bowl in your steamer basket.
4. Pour 1 cup of water into your Instant Pot. Lower the basket into your Instant Pot.
5. Seal and cook on low pressure for 7 minutes. Depressurize quickly.
6. Stir well and allow to rest, it will finish cooking in its own heat.

THAI EGGS

Prep time: 15 minutes
Cooking time: 7 minutes
Nutrition per serving:

Setting: Steam
Serves: 2

Calories: 125   Sugar: 2   Protein: 16

Carbs: 5   Fat: 9   GL: 1

Ingredients:

- 3 eggs
- 1/4 cup of milk
- 1tsp Thai curry paste
- 1 shredded cooked onion
- 1tsp minced garlic

Recipe:

1. Spray a heat-proof bowl that fits in your Instant Pot with nonstick spray.
2. Whisk together the eggs, milk, paste, and garlic.
3. Pour into the bowl. Add the onion.
4. Place the bowl in your steamer basket.
5. Pour 1 cup of water into your Instant Pot.
6. Lower the basket into your Instant Pot.
7. Seal and cook on low pressure for 7 minutes.
8. Depressurize quickly.
9. Stir well and allow to rest, it will finish cooking in its own heat.

ALMOND FLAKE "OATS"

Prep time: 10 minutes   **Setting:** Manual

Cooking time: 5 minutes   **Serves:** 2

Nutrition per serving:

Calories: 380   Sugar: 1   Protein: 15

Carbs: 11   Fat: 18   GL: 4

Ingredients:

- 0.5 cup mashed flaked almonds
- 2 cups milk
- 2tbsp powdered sweetener
- 1tbsp cinnamon
- 1tsp nutmeg

Recipe:

1. Pour the milk into your Instant Pot.
2. Add the remaining ingredients, stir well. Seal and close the vent.
3. Choose Manual and set to cook 5 minutes.
4. Release the pressure naturally.

BERRY OATS

Prep time: 10 minutes
Cooking time: 5 minutes

Setting: Manual
Serves: 2

Nutrition per serving:

Calories: 250

Sugar: 5

Protein: 6

Carbs: 19

Fat: 5

GL: 9

Ingredients:

- 0.5 cup high fiber steel cut oats
- 2 cups milk
- 1 cup mixed berries

Recipe:

1. Pour the milk into your Instant Pot.
2. Add the oats, stir well.
3. Seal and close the vent.
4. Choose Manual and set to cook 5 minutes.
5. Release the pressure naturally.
6. Stir in the berries.

SWEET CHILI EGGS

Prep time: 15 minutes
Cooking time: 7 minutes

Setting: Steam
Serves: 2

Nutrition per serving:

Calories: 165

Fat: 11

Carbs: 6

Protein: 19

Sugar: 0

GL: 2

Ingredients:

- 3 eggs
- 1/4 cup of milk
- 1/4 cup cooked sausage
- 2tbsp sugar-free sweet chili sauce

Recipe:

1. Spray a heat-proof bowl that fits in your Instant Pot with nonstick spray.
2. Whisk together the eggs, milk, and sauce.
3. Pour into the bowl. Add the sausage.

4. Place the bowl in your steamer basket. Pour 1 cup of water into your Instant Pot.
5. Lower the basket into your Instant Pot.
6. Seal and cook on low pressure for 7 minutes. Depressurize quickly.
7. Stir well and allow to rest, it will finish cooking in its own heat.

EGGS WITH SPINACH

Prep time: 15 minutes   **Setting:** Steam
Cooking time: 7 minutes   **Serves:** 2
Nutrition per serving:

Calories: 110	Sugar: 0	Protein: 16
Carbs: 4	Fat: 8	GL: 1

Ingredients:
- 3 eggs
- 2 cups spinach
- 1/4 cup of milk
- 2tbsp grated Parmesan
- pinch of salt

Recipe:
1. Spray a heat-proof bowl that fits in your Instant Pot with nonstick spray.
2. Whisk together the eggs, milk, and salt. Pour into the bowl.
3. Place the bowl in your steamer basket. Pour 1 cup of water into your Instant Pot.
4. Lower the basket into your Instant Pot.
5. Seal and cook on low pressure for 7 minutes.
6. Depressurize quickly. Stir in the spinach and Parmesan.
7. Stir well and allow to rest, it will finish cooking in its own heat.

INSTANT POT PULLED PORK

Cooking Time: 65 Minutes   **Yield: 5 Servings**
Ingredients

2 tablespoons of stevia   1 teaspoon of red chili powder
2 tablespoons of smoked paprika   3.5 pounds of pork shoulder
Salt and black pepper, to taste   3 cups of chicken broth

Directions

1. Combine smoked paprika, chili powder, salt, black pepper, and stevia in a bowl.
2. Rub the pork shoulder with the spices. Pour broth into the instant pot.
3. Place pork in the pot and lock the lid. Set the knob to the sealing position.
4. Set the timer to 45 minutes at high pressure.
5. Once timer beeps, release the steam naturally for 10 minutes, followed by quick release.
6. Open the pot and then remove the meat. Use a fork to shred the meat.
7. Sprinkle some additional spice rub on top of meat if preferred. Mix well and serve.

TOFU SCRAMBLE WITH VEG

Prep time: 15 minutes   **Setting:** Steam
Cooking time: 7 minutes   **Serves:** 2
Nutrition per serving:

Calories:	Sugar: 2	Protein: 18
Carbs: 7	Fat: 3	GL: 2

Ingredients:
- 1 cup firm silken tofu
- 1 cup mixed diced vegetables
- 1tsp mixed herbs
- pinch of salt

Recipe:

1. Spray a heat-proof bowl that fits in your Instant Pot with nonstick spray.
2. Roughly chop the tofu. Mix in the other ingredients. Pour into the bowl.
3. Place the bowl in your steamer basket.
4. Pour 1 cup of water into your Instant Pot. Lower the basket into your Instant Pot.
5. Seal and cook on low pressure for 7 minutes. Depressurize quickly.
6. Stir well and allow to rest, it will finish cooking in its own heat.

SPAGHETTI SQUASH IN AN INSTANT POT

Cooking Time: 15 Minutes   Yield: 4 Servings

Ingredients

2 pounds of spaghetti squash

1 cup of water

2 cups cooked and grounded beef

Directions

1. Pierce the squash using a paring knife. Pour water about one cup in the instant pot
2. Adjust steamer basket inside the instant pot.
3. Place the squash onto the steamer basket and lock the instant pot.
4. Set the timer to 15 minutes at high pressure. Once the time completes, release the steam naturally. Carefully open the instant pot and remove the squash.
5. Cool and then shred the squash with a fork. Let it get cool for 10 minutes before serving.
6. Serve with grounded beef

CHEESY EGG BAKE

Cooking Time: 7 Minutes   Yield: 2 Servings

Ingredients

4 slices bacon, chopped

6 eggs

¼ cup of coconut milk

½ cup shredded cheddar cheese

Salt and black pepper, to taste

1 green onion, chopped

Directions

1. Turn on the sauté mode of the instant pot and cook bacon until crisp.
2. Transfer the bacon to plate for further use. Then add chopped onions and sauté until tender. In a bowl, whisk eggs with cheese and coconut milk.
3. Sprinkle salt and black pepper and add green onions and bacon.
4. Pour the mixture into the oil greased pan that fits inside the instant pot.

5. Pour 1 cup of water in the instant pot. Set the trivet on top.
6. Place the pan on top of the trivet.
7. Lock the lid and set the timer to 5 minutes, at high pressure.
8. Once the timer beeps, release the steam naturally and take out the pan. Serve.

INSTANT POT CRANBERRY MEATBALLS

Cooking Time: 20 Minutes   **Yield: 2 Servings**

Ingredients

1 tablespoon olive oil
10 frozen meatballs
½ cup beef broth
12 ounces cranberry sauce

1 teaspoon garlic powder
1 tablespoon dried minced onions

Directions

1. Pour oil in the instant pot and add meatballs to the pot. Cook for 5 minutes.
2. Pour broth around the meatballs.
3. Then add cranberry sauce, minced onions, and garlic powder. Lok the instant pot lid.
4. Set the timer to 5 minutes at high pressure. Afterward, release the steam naturally.
5. Open the pot and transfer the meatball to a baking sheet. Broil in oven for 10 minutes.
6. Meanwhile, turn on the sauté mode of instant pot and thicken the sauce for 5 minutes.
7. Once done serve. Enjoy.

SALMON WITH GINGER SAUCE

Cooking Time: 9 Minutes   **Yield: 2 Servings**

Ingredients

1.5 pound salmon
1 tablespoon white vinegar
2 teaspoons minced ginger

1 teaspoon minced garlic
Salt and pepper, to taste
2 tablespoons stevia

Directions

1. In a bowl, combine stevia, ginger, garlic, salt, and black pepper. Then add the vinegar.
2. Now rub the salmon with the bowl mixture. Allow the seafood to marinate for 20 minutes.
3. Pour 2 cups of water in the instant pot. Place steaming rack on into the instant pot.
4. Cover the steaming rack with a sling of aluminum foil.
5. Place salmon on the steaming rack with the sauce. Cook on low for 4 minutes.
6. Once timer beeps, quick release the steam. Open the instant pot.
7. Take out the aluminum foil and place it on a baking sheet.
8. Broil the salmon in the oven by placing it in oil greased baking sheet for 5 minutes at 350 degrees F. Once done, serve. Enjoy.

PICNIC CHICKEN STEW

Cooking Time: 20 Minutes   **Yield: 4 Servings**
Ingredients
8 chicken breasts   Salt and black pepper, to taste
16 ounces of diced tomatoes   ½ cup of beef broth
3 minced garlic cloves   6 tablespoons of oil
Directions
1. Turn on sauté mode of the instant pot and add oil and garlic. Cook until aroma comes.
2. Then add breasts and sear for 3 minutes. Next, add salt, pepper, broth, and diced tomatoes.
3. Lock the lid and set the timer to 15-20 minutes at high pressure.
4. Once timer beeps, release the steam quickly. Stir and enjoy.

BEEF WITH DRIED APRICOTS

Cooking Time: 60 Minutes   **Yield: 4 Servings**
Ingredients
2 cups dried apricots   1 teaspoon coriander, ground
2 teaspoons garlic powder   3 cups beef stock
Salt and black pepper, to taste   2.5 pounds beef brisket, boneless

Directions

1. Dump the listed ingredients in the instant pot.
2. Press meat stew button and cook on high for 60 minutes. Once timer beeps, release steam naturally for 15 minutes. Open the pot and stir. Serve.

CHICKEN IN BEST GRAVY

Cooking Time: 15 Minutes   **Yield: 4 Servings**

Ingredients

2.5 pounds of boneless chicken leg

2 tablespoons of tomato paste

4 cloves garlic, crushed

Salt and freshly ground black pepper, to taste

2 teaspoons of ginger, grated

½ cup coconut amino

Directions

1. Dump all the ingredients inside the instant pot. Lock the lid and set the timer to 15 minutes at high pressure. Once timer beeps, release the steam quickly.
2. Open the pot and then stir the ingredients. Once done, serve and enjoy.

SIRLOIN STEAK WITH ONION GRAVY MIX

Cooking Time: 24 Minutes   **Yield: 3 Servings**

Ingredients

2 pounds sirloin steak, sliced

Salt and black pepper, to taste

6 tablespoons of onion gravy mix

1/3 cup Almond flour, for dredging

1 can cream of mushroom soup

2 cups beef bone broth

2 tablespoons of olive oil

Directions

1. First, rub the steak with salt and black pepper.
2. Dredge the steak in almond flour and then set aside for further use.
3. Pour oil in the instant pot. Cook the steak in the pot for 2 minutes each side.

4. Open the pot and then add cream of mushroom soup, onion gravy mix, and broth.
5. Lock the lid and cook it for 20 minutes at high pressure.
6. Then release the steam naturally for 12 minutes. Serve hot. Enjoy.

QUICK BROWN GRAVY BEEF ROAST

Cooking Time: 40 Minutes   **Yield: 4 Servings**
Ingredients
2.5-3 pounds beef roast   1 cup heavy cream
4 tablespoons salad dressing mix,   1 cup of water
dried Italian
Directions
1. Dump the ingredients in the instant pot and set the timer to 30 minutes at high pressure.
2. Once the timer beeps, release the steam naturally for 10 minutes, followed by quick release.
3. Take out the beef roast and place it on a greased baking sheet.
4. Then place in oven and broil for 10 minutes at 375 degrees F.
5. Meanwhile, sauté the sauce inside the instant pot and reduce to ¼ of the amount.
6. Serve the sauce with the roast.

YUMMY EGG AND SPINACH CASSEROLE

Cooking Time: 12 Minutes   **Yield: 2 Servings**
Ingredients
4 tablespoons olive oil   1/3 cup baby spinach, washed
1/3 cup pork Sausage, cooked   and chopped
and chopped   1/3 cup leeks, chopped
8 organic Eggs, whisked   Salt and black pepper, to taste
1 tablespoon of garlic, minced
Directions
1. Turn on the sauté mode of the instant pot. Add the oil to the instant pot and turn on the sauté mode. Put the leeks and spinach in the pot and cook for 2 minutes.

2. Remove the vegetables from the pot. Then add the garlic and cook until the aroma comes.
3. In a bowl, whisk the eggs along with sausage.
4. Add garlic from the instant pot to the egg mixture.
5. Then add spinach and leeks and season it with salt and black pepper. Mix ingredients well.
6. Pour 2 cups of water in the pot and place trivet on top.
7. Make a sling of aluminum foil and place on a trivet. Place egg bowl on a trivet.
8. Set the timer to 10 minutes after locking the lid.
9. Once the timer beeps, release the steam naturally, followed by quick release steam.
10. Cut the casserole into slices and serve. Enjoy.

CLASSIC BREAKFAST CUPS WITH MUSHROOM AND TURKEY BACON

Cooking Time: 5 Minutes   **Yield: 1 Serving**

Ingredients

3 organic eggs

16 medium slices of turkey bacon

2 broccoli florets, chopped

4 mushrooms, chopped

Sea Salt and black pepper, to taste

Directions

1. Pour one cup of water in the instant pot. Set the trivet in the instant pot.
2. Now grease two ramekins with oil spray.
3. In a bowl, whisk eggs and then add salt, black pepper, mushroom, broccoli florets, and turkey bacon. Mix the egg mixture well.
4. Divide the egg mixture between ramekins.
5. Place ramekin on a trivet and lock the lid of the instant pot.
6. Select the timer manually for 5 minutes at high pressure.
7. When the timer beeps, quick release the steam.
8. Open the pot and remove ramekins. Serve and enjoy.

EGGS WITH BLACK OLIVES

Cooking Time: 5 Minutes   **Yield: 1 Serving**

Ingredients

Salt and pepper, to taste
2 organic eggs
2 tablespoons of soy milk

1 cup black olives, chopped
½ tablespoon of lard, melted
Oil spray, for greasing

Directions

1. Pour one cup of water in the instant pot. Set the trivet in the instant pot.
2. Grease a small heat-proof pan and set aside. Add eggs in the bowl and whisk.
3. Add the lard, soy milk, black olive, black pepper, and salt.
4. Whisk all the ingredients well. Pour the batter to the heatproof pan. Place the heatproof pan on the trivet. Lock the instant pot lid and set time to 5 minutes at high pressure.
5. Once timer beeps, naturally release steam. Take out the heatproof pan and serve the eggs.

COCONUT CABBAGE MIX

Cooking Time: 5 Minutes   **Yield: 1 Serving**

Ingredients

4 tablespoons of coconut oil
1 small onion, sliced
Salt and black pepper, to taste
½ teaspoon of garlic, minced

1 -1/2 cups cabbage, sliced
1/3 cup coconut milk, unsweetened

Directions

1. Turn on the sauté mode. Add coconut oil to the instant pot and let it get hot.
2. Add onions and cook until translucent. Next, add salt, black pepper, garlic, and cook.
3. Then add cabbage and ¼ amount of coconut milk, and cook for 1 minute.
4. Lock the lid and set the timer to 2 minutes at low pressure.
5. After 2 minutes quick release the steam.
6. Then press the keep warm button and pour the remaining coconut milk.
7. Stir for 4 minutes. Serve hot and enjoy.

BRUSSELS SPROUTS AND CELERY STEW

Cooking Time: 13 Minutes   Yield: 1 Serving

Ingredients

2 cups beef broth

1 cup Brussels sprouts

1 white onion, chopped

1 cup celery, sliced

1 cup coconut milk, divided

Salt and pepper, to taste

Directions

1. Combine all the listed ingredients in the instant Pot and lock the lid.
2. Set timer to 10 minutes. Once the timer beeps, quick release the steam.
3. Now turn it off and press the sauté mode. Let it get thickened. Once it's done serve.

5 INGREDIENTS GARDEN STEW

Cooking Time: 10 Minutes   Yield: 2-3 Serving

Ingredients

6 cups beef broth

4 tablespoons of olive oil

2 small zucchinis, sliced

Salt and pepper, to taste

6 ounces of Shiitake mushrooms, chopped

4 cloves garlic, minced

4 teaspoons, dried savory leaves

Directions

Combine all the ingredients in the instant pot. Lock the lid and set the timer to 10 minutes at high pressure. Once timer beeps, quick release the steam. Serve.

RASPBERRY, STRAWBERRY, AND RHUBARB COMPOTE

Cooking Time: 10 Minutes   Yield: 3 Servings

Ingredients

1 pound strawberries

1 pound rhubarb

½ pound of raspberries

½ cup stevia, or to taste

½ cup of lime juice

Directions

Dump all the ingredients in the instant pot. Set timer for 10 minutes at high pressure.
Once timer beeps, release the steam quickly. Open the pot and stir.
Serve.

Low Carb Lunches And Dinners

When it comes to our lunch or dinner, it is generally much easier to avoid eating only carbs. After all, we have a wide range of proteins and vegetables that we enjoy eating around this time of day. However you might be finding it difficult to throw together a filling main meal without adding a side of carbs. To combat this, all the meals in this chapter come with a side of a low carb alternative.

LOW CARB PUMPKIN PIE PUDDING

Cooking Time: 20 Minutes   **Yield: 2 Servings**
Ingredients
3 eggs, whisked   16 ounces of pumpkin puree
1/3 cup of almond milk, whipping   2 teaspoons pumpkin pie spice
¼ cup of stevia sweetener
Directions
1. In a bowl, whisk eggs and add almond milk, stevia, pumpkin puree, and pumpkin pie spice.
2. Grease the oil in a steel pan and then pour egg mixture in it.
3. Pour 2 cups of water inside the instant pot and set trivet in the pot.
4. Place steel pan on top of the trivet. Cover the pan with the aluminum foil.
5. Close the pot and set the timer to 20 minutes at high pressure.
6. Once timer beeps, quick release the steam. Remove the lid of the instant pot.
7. Chill for 2 hours and then serve with whipping cream.

ITALIAN BEEF ROAST

Cooking Time: 70 Minutes   **Yield: 5 Servings**
Ingredients
4 pounds of beef roast   4 tablespoons of garlic infused
2 tablespoons of red pepper   olive oil

Salt and black pepper, to taste   1 cup beef broth
20 ounces of Peperoncini
Directions
1. Take a plastic bag and place beef roast, red pepper, garlic infused oil, salt, and black pepper in it. Let it marinate for 30 minutes.
2. After marinating, add beef, a jar of the peperoncini and broth into the instant pot.
3. Set timer for 70 minutes at high pressure.
4. After 70 minutes, naturally, release the steam for 20 minutes.
5. Serve Beef in bowls and enjoy.

RED CABBAGE MIX

Cooking Time: 5 Minutes   **Yield: 3 Servings**
Ingredients
4 tablespoons of coconut oil   6 cups of red cabbage,
1 teaspoon of butter   shredded
2 garlic cloves   Salt and black pepper to taste
                                                         1/3 cup of water

Directions
1. Turn on the sauté mode of the instant pot. Add coconut oil and butter to the instant pot.
2. Heat the butter to let it melt. Add salt, pepper, and garlic cloves.
3. Cook until aroma comes. Add cabbage and pour water.
4. Lock the lid and set the timer to 5 minutes.
5. Once timer beeps, release the steam naturally. Serve and enjoy.

IRISH LAMB STEW

Cooking Time: 45 Minutes   **Yield: 4 Servings**
Ingredients
2 pounds of lamb shank   ½ cup of green beans,
3 cups of chicken broth   chopped
1 green onion   Salt and black pepper
¼ teaspoon of thyme   2 tablespoons of olive oil
Directions

1. Turn on sauté mode of instant pot and add olive oil.
2. Sear the meat for 3 minutes in oil from both the sides.
3. Add green beans, green onion, and cook for one minute at sautéing mode.
4. Sprinkle salt and black pepper. Pour broth and add thyme to the pot.
5. Turn off the sauté mode and then set the timer to 45 minutes at high pressure.
6. Once timer beeps, release the steam naturally.
7. Open the instant pot and stir the mixture. Then serve.

BLUEBERRY AND STRAWBERRY JAM

Cooking Time: 3 Minutes   **Yield: 4 Servings**
Ingredients

1 pound of diced organic blueberries

½ pound strawberries

¼ cup of strawberry juice

1 cup stevia

Directions

1. Turn on the sauté mode the instant pot. Sauté for a few seconds and add stevia.
2. Then add the strawberry juice, strawberries, and blueberries.
3. When the mixture started to bubble lock the lid of the pot.
4. Set manual setting for 3 minutes at high pressure.
5. Once timer beeps, quick release the steam. Remove the lid of the instant pot.
6. Turn on the sauté mode, and boil the excess liquid.
7. Pour the jam to the container and the seal tight. Serve or store for further use.

VEGETABLES IN HALF AND HALF

Cooking Time: 8 Minutes   **Yield: 2 Servings**
Ingredients

2 medium parsnips, peeled and cubed

1 fennel bulb, sliced

3 cloves garlic, minced

1 cup chicken broth
1 cup half-and-half

Salt and pepper, to taste

Directions
1. Add fennel bulbs, parsnip, chicken broth, garlic, salt, and pepper into the instant pot.
2. Lock the lid of the pot. Set timer for 5 minutes at high pressure.
3. Once time beeps, quick release the steam. Turn on the sauté mode and reduce the liquid.
4. Stir occasionally. Next, add half and half and mix well.
5. Stir for 2 more minutes and then serve the dish hot. Enjoy.

CHEDDAR AND MUSTARD SAUCE

Cooking Time: 4 Minutes   **Yield: 4 Servings**

Ingredients
4 tablespoons of butter
1 small onion, chopped
2 cups almond milk

4 ounces of cheddar cheese
1 teaspoon of dry mustard
Salt and black, pepper

Directions
1. Turn on sauté mode of the instant pot and melt butter in it. Now add onion and cook for one minute. Gradually pour in the milk and start whisking it.
2. Stir and cook until thickened. Then add cheese and dry mustard. Lock the lid.
3. Set timer for 2 minutes at low. Afterward, release the steam quickly.
4. Add salt, pepper. Stir to mix all the ingredients. Serve and enjoy.

CREAMY BROCCOLI AND HAM

Cooking Time: 10 Minutes   **Yield: 4 Servings**

Ingredients
20 ounces of broccoli
12 ounces of ham, smoked and chopped
8 ounces of fat-free cream of mushroom soup

1 cup almond milk
2 cups of Cheddar cheese, shredded
Salt and black pepper
2 teaspoons of olive oil

Directions
1. Turn on the sauté mode of the instant pot. Add oil and heat it.
2. Then add broccoli and cook for one minute. Next, add ham and season it with salt and pepper. Pour in the cream of mushroom soup and almond milk and lock the lid.
3. Set timer for 4 minutes at high pressure. Once timer beeps, quick release the steam.
4. Reduce the liquid by turning on the sauté mode. Keep stirring.
5. After a few mins, add cheese and cook for 2 minutes at sauté mode. Once it's done serve.

GLAZED CARROTS AND CAULIFLOWER

Cooking Time: 5 Minutes   **Yields: 2 Servings**
Ingredients
1/3 pound of baby carrot
1 cauliflower head, small and chopped
3/4 cup lime juice

3 tablespoons butter/olive oil
1/3 cup stevia
1/4 teaspoon ground cinnamon
Salt and black pepper, to taste

Directions
1. Combine all the ingredients in the instant pot. Lock the lid and set the timer to 5 minutes.
2. Open timer beeps, release the steam quickly. Open the instant pot lid. Stir and serve.

BROTH-BRAISED CABBAGE

Cooking Time: 5 Minutes   **Yield: 2 Servings**
Ingredients
1 head of cabbage, sliced
1 small onion
2 garlic cloves, minced
1/3 teaspoon star anise seeds

1/4 cup vegetable broth
2 slices of diced bacon
2 teaspoons of olive oil
Salt and black pepper, to taste

Directions
1. Turn on sauté mode of the instant pot. Add oil and heat it.
2. Then add bacon and cook until crisp.

3. Then add small onions and garlic cloves and cook until aroma comes.
4. Add salt, pepper and anise seed. At the end add cabbage and pour the broth.
5. Cook on high for 3 minutes. Then quickly release the steam.
6. Serve and enjoy.

SHREDDED BBQ CREAM CHEESE CHICKEN

Cooking Time: 13 Minutes   Yield: 2 Servings
Ingredients

2 pounds of chicken breast   ½ cup of BBQ sauce, Keto based
1 cup of water   6 ounces of cream cheese

Directions

1. Pour water in instant pot. Add chicken, and lock the lid.
2. Set timer for 12 minutes at high pressure. Once timer beeps, quick release the steam.
3. Transfer the chicken from the instant pot and place it on the cutting board.
4. Use a fork to shred the chicken meat. Drain water from the instant pot.
5. Transfer the shredded chicken back to the pot.
6. Next, add cream cheese, and BBQ sauce. Stir and combine all the ingredients.
7. Turn on sauté mode and then cook for one minute. Serve and enjoy.

RANCH DUMP STYLE PORK CHOPS

Cooking Time: 12 Minutes   Yield: 6 Servings
Ingredients

4 pounds of pork chops   18 ounces of cream of chicken
2 ounces of ranch dressing mix   soup
                                         2 cups of water

Directions

Combine the listed ingredients in the instant pot. Lock the lid of the instant pot and set the timer to 12 minutes at high pressure. Once timer beeps, naturally release the steam for 12 minutes. Then quickly release the steam. Open the pot, stir the ingredients and then serve.

INSTANT POT CINNAMON APRICOT AND PEARS

Cooking Time: 5 Minutes   **Yield: 3 Servings**

Ingredients

¼ cup of lime juice

2 apricot peeled

1 teaspoon of cinnamon

2 pears, peeled

Salt, pinch

2 scoops of stevia powder

Directions

1. Peel, core, and slice the fruits. Transfer the apricot, cinnamon, pears, salt, and stevia in the instant pot. Pour the lime juice in the instant pot.
2. Lock the lid of the instant pot, and set the timer to 2 minutes at high pressure.
3. Once timer beeps, release the steam quickly. Turn on the sauté mode and reduce the liquid.
4. Serve immediately and enjoy.

BEETS DIJON

Cooking Time: 14 Minutes   **Yield: 2 Servings**

Ingredients

1 pound beets, peeled, cubed (1/2-inch)

1/3 cup finely chopped onion

1/3 cup sour cream

2 tablespoons Dijon mustard

2–3 teaspoons lemon juice

Salt and white pepper, to taste

Directions

1. Combine beets, onions, Dijon mustard, lemon juice, salt, and black pepper in a bowl and set aside. Pour water in the instant pot and set trivet inside the pot.
2. Place the heatproof bowl, having beets on a trivet and lock the lid.

3. Set timer to 12 minutes. Once timer beeps, release the steam quickly.
4. Remove the beets bowl from the instant pot. Drain water from pot and turn on sauté mode.
5. Transfer beet to the pot and add sour cream. Cook for 2 minutes and then serve.

CHOCOLATE FONDUE WITH STRAWBERRIES

Cooking Time: 7 Minutes   **Yield: 6 Servings**
Ingredients
3 cups dark chocolate   1 teaspoon of ginger syrup
1.5 cup heavy cream   2 tablespoons of lime juice
1 teaspoon of coconut oil   Dippers: 2 cups of strawberries
Directions
1. Transfer coconut oil, chocolate, lime juice, ginger syrup and cream in a heatproof bowl.
2. Pour 2 cups of water in the pot. Adjust bowl inside the pot.
3. Now, turn on sauté mode and cook the ingredients to the bowl until combined and mixed well. Lock the lid and set the timer to 2 minutes at high pressure.
4. Then quickly release the steam.
5. Once thickened, serve the chocolate fondue instantly with strawberry.

NUTS AND PEARS COMPOTE

Cooking Time: 5 Minutes   **Yield: 4 Servings**
Ingredients
2 ounces of almond, chopped   6 ounces of Pears, peeled and
6 ounces of hazelnuts   chopped
2 ounces of cashews   ½ cup lime juice
                                  1/8 teaspoon salt

Directions
Combine all ingredients in instant pot. Lock the lid and set the timer to 5 minutes. Once timer beeps, quick release the steam. Serve warm.

GREEN BEAN CASSEROLE

Cooking Time: 20 Minutes   **Yield: 3 Servings**

Ingredients

1 can of cream of mushroom soup

1 cup sour cream, full fat

12 ounces of green beans, thawed

Salt and black pepper, to taste

2 green onions, chopped

1 teaspoon of olive oil

1 cup parmesan cheese, grated

Directions

1. Turn on the sauté mode of instant pot and add oil, and green onions. Cook unit aroma comes.   Next, add green beans and cook for one minute.
2. Now add cream of mushroom soup.   Lok the lid of the instant pot.
3. Set timer for 12 minutes at high. Once timer beeps, do quick release steam.
4. Season the green beans with salt and black pepper and add sour cream.
5. Stir and serve hot with garnish of parmesan cheese.
6. Broil cheese for 5 minutes before serving. Enjoy.

PLAIN MEAT LOAF

Cooking Time: 30 Minutes   **Yield: 3 Servings**

Ingredients

2 pounds beef lean and ground

½ cup almond milk

2 eggs

1/3 cup chopped onion

1 teaspoon of Italian seasoning

Salt and black pepper, to taste

Directions

1. Place a steamer rack inside the instant pot and pour two cups of water.
2. Mix all the listed ingredients in a bowl with hands. Make a large loaf of the mixture.
3. Now place meatloaf over an aluminum foil and wrap the meatloaf in the foil.

4. Place foil on the steaming rack.
5. Lock the lid of the instant pot and set the timer to 30 minutes at high pressure.
6. Once timer beeps, do a natural release for 10 minutes, followed by quick release.
7. Remove the meatloaf from the foil. Transfer it to cutting board, and cut into slices.
8. Serve with your favorite dipping sauce.

LEMONY DIJON MEAT LOAF

Cooking Time: 35 Minutes   Yield: 3-4 Servings
Main Ingredients

2 pounds lean ground beef
1 cup almond meal
2 eggs
1 tablespoon lemon, zest, and juice

2 teaspoons Dijon mustard
Seasoning Salt and black pepper, to taste

Directions
Pour 1-1/2 cups of water and place trivet inside the instant pot.
1. Mix all the listed ingredients in a mixing bowl. Make a large loaf of the meat mixture.
2. Now place meatloaf over an aluminum foil and wrap the meat in foil.
3. Place foil on the trivet.
4. Lock the lid of the instant Pot and set a timer to 35 minutes at high pressure.
5. Once timer beeps, do a natural release for 15 minutes, followed by quick release.
6. Remove the meatloaf from the foil.
7. Transfer to cutting board, and cut into slices after letting it get cold. Serve.

GREEK-STYLE GREEN BEANS

Cooking Time: 12 Minutes   Yield: 3 Servings

Ingredients

1 pound green beans

26 ounces of fresh tomatoes, diced

1 onion, chopped

2 tablespoons of olive oil

2 garlic cloves

1/3 cup of water

Salt and pepper, to taste

Directions

1. Turn on the sauté mode of the instant pot. Add onions and olive oil.
2. Cook onions until translucent. Add garlic and cook until aroma comes.
3. Next, add diced tomatoes and sauté it for 2 minutes.
4. Now, add green beans, salt, and pepper. Add water and lock the lid.
5. Set timer for 10 minutes at high. Once timer beeps, release the steam quickly.
6. Open the pot and stir the ingredients. Serve.

ITALIAN TOFU SCRAMBLE

Prep time: 15 minutes

Cooking time: 7 minutes

Setting: Steam

Serves: 2

Nutrition per serving:

Calories: 210	Sugar: 4	Protein: 18
Carbs: 9	Fat: 3	GL: 4

Ingredients:

- 1 cup firm silken tofu
- 1 cup chopped cherry tomatoes
- 1 cup mixed chopped squash
- 1tsp mixed herbs
- pinch of salt

Recipe:

1. Spray a heat-proof bowl that fits in your Instant Pot with nonstick spray.
2. Chop the tofu finely.
3. Mix with the other ingredients.
4. Pour into the bowl.
5. Place the bowl in your steamer basket.
6. Pour 1 cup of water into your Instant Pot.
7. Lower the basket into your Instant Pot.

8. Seal and cook on low pressure for 7 minutes.
9. Depressurize quickly.
10.   Stir well and allow to rest, it will finish cooking in its own heat.

KALE SAUSAGE STEW

Prep time: 15 minutes
Cooking time: 10 minutes
Setting: Stew
Serves: 2
Nutrition per serving:

Calories: 300   Sugar: 1   Protein: 30
Carbs: 9   Fat: 20   GL: 3

Ingredients:
- 1lb cooked chopped sausage
- 1lb shredded kale
- 1 cup vegetable broth
- 1tbsp mixed herbs
- 1tbsp gravy

Recipe:
1. Mix all the ingredients in your Instant Pot.
2. Cook on Stew for 10 minutes.
3. Release the pressure naturally.

TOMATO AND BROCCOLI

Prep time: 15 minutes
Cooking time: 10 minutes
Setting: Stew
Serves: 2
Nutrition per serving:

Calories: 130   Sugar: 3   Protein: 6
Carbs: 6   Fat: 10   GL: 2

Ingredients:
- 1lb chopped broccoli
- 1lb cherry tomato
- 1 cup low sodium broth
- 1tbsp dry basil
- 1 minced onion

Recipe:

1. Mix all the ingredients in your Instant Pot.
2. Cook on Stew for 10 minutes.
3. Release the pressure naturally.

MUSHROOM TOFU STEW

Prep time: 15 minutes
Cooking time: 10 minutes
Nutrition per serving:

Setting: Stew
Serves: 2

Calories: 180
Carbs: 5

Sugar: 1
Fat: 11

Protein: 34
GL: 2

Ingredients:
- 1lb chopped mushrooms
- 1lb chopped tofu
- 1 cup mushroom soup
- 1tbsp mixed herbs
- 1 minced onion

Recipe:
1. Mix all the ingredients in your Instant Pot.
2. Cook on Stew for 10 minutes.
3. Release the pressure naturally.

EGG AND CHICKEN STEW

Prep time: 15 minutes
Cooking time: 10 minutes
Nutrition per serving:

Setting: Stew
Serves: 2

Calories: 340
Carbs: 10

Sugar: 2
Fat: 20

Protein: 43
GL: 7

Ingredients:
- 1lb cooked shredded chicken
- 1lb chopped vegetables
- 1 cup low sodium broth
- 2 hard boiled eggs, quartered
- 1tbsp mixed herbs

Recipe:

1. Mix all the ingredients in your Instant Pot.
2. Cook on Stew for 10 minutes.
3. Release the pressure naturally.

SHRIMP CHOWDER

Prep time: 15 minutes   **Setting:** Stew
Cooking time: 10 minutes   **Serves:** 2
Nutrition per serving:
Calories: 270   Sugar: 3   Protein: 35
Carbs: 10   Fat: 15   GL: 8
Ingredients:
- 1lb cooked shrimp
- 1lb chopped vegetables
- 1 cup white sauce
- 1tbsp mixed herbs

Recipe:
1. Mix all the ingredients in your Instant Pot.
2. Cook on Stew for 10 minutes.
3. Release the pressure naturally.

PUMPKIN SOUP

Prep time: 15 minutes   **Setting:** Stew
Cooking time: 10 minutes   **Serves:** 2
Nutrition per serving:
Calories: 200   Sugar: 2   Protein: 2
Carbs: 7   Fat: 11   GL: 2
Ingredients:
- 1lb chopped pumpkin
- 1lb chopped tomato
- 1 cup broth
- 1tbsp mixed herbs
- 1 minced onion

Recipe:
1. Mix all the ingredients in your Instant Pot.

2. Cook on Stew for 10 minutes.
3. Release the pressure naturally.
4. Blend.

IRISH LAMB

Prep time: 15 minutes   **Setting:** Stew
Cooking time: 10 minutes   **Serves:** 2
Nutrition per serving:
Calories: 450   Sugar: 4   Protein: 41
Carbs: 10   Fat: 27   GL: 9
Ingredients:
- 1lb cooked chopped lamb
- 1lb shredded cabbage
- 1 cup low carb beer
- 1tbsp mixed herbs
- 1 minced onion

Recipe:
1. Mix all the ingredients in your Instant Pot.
2. Cook on Stew for 10 minutes.
3. Release the pressure naturally.

CLAM CHOWDER

Prep time: 15 minutes   **Setting:** Stew
Cooking time: 10 minutes   **Serves:** 2
Nutrition per serving:
Calories: 300   Sugar: 3   Protein: 42
Carbs: 4   Fat: 3   GL: 2
Ingredients:
- 1lb cooked shelled clams
- 1lb chopped vegetables
- 1 cup white sauce
- 1tbsp mixed herbs
- 1 minced onion

Recipe:
1. Mix all the ingredients in your Instant Pot.

2. Cook on Stew for 10 minutes.
3. Release the pressure naturally.

EGGS AND SAUSAGE

Prep time: 15 minutes   **Setting:** Steam
Cooking time: 7 minutes   **Serves:** 2
Nutrition per serving:

Calories: 210	Sugar: 0	Protein: 22
Carbs: 3	Fat: 15	GL: 1

Ingredients:
- 3 eggs
- 1/4 cup of milk
- 1 cup chopped cooked sausage
- 0.5 cup chopped cooked bacon
- pinch of salt

Recipe:
1. Spray a heat-proof bowl that fits in your Instant Pot with nonstick spray.
2. Whisk together the eggs, milk, and salt.
3. Pour into the bowl. Add the sausage and bacon.
4. Place the bowl in your steamer basket. Pour 1 cup of water into your Instant Pot.
5. Lower the basket into your Instant Pot.
6. Seal and cook on low pressure for 7 minutes. Depressurize quickly.
7. Stir well and allow to rest, it will finish cooking in its own heat.

PORK AND MUSHROOMS

Prep time: 15 minutes   **Setting:** Stew
Cooking time: 10 minutes   **Serves:** 2
Nutrition per serving:

Calories: 410	Carbs: 10	Sugar: 1

Fat: 20   Protein: 42   GL: 8

Ingredients:
- 1lb cooked diced pork
- 1lb chopped mixed mushrooms
- 1 cup mushroom soup
- 1tbsp mixed herbs
- 1tbsp shredded cheddar

Recipe:
1. Mix all the ingredients in your Instant Pot.
2. Cook on Stew for 10 minutes.
3. Release the pressure naturally.

CHICKEN AND TOMATO STEW

Prep time: 15 minutes   **Setting:** Stew
Cooking time: 10 minutes   **Serves:** 2
Nutrition per serving:
Calories: 230   Sugar: 2   Protein: 42
Carbs: 6   Fat: 13   GL: 4

Ingredients:
- 1lb cooked diced chicken
- 1lb chopped tomatoes
- 1 cup vegetable broth
- 1tbsp mixed herbs
- 1 minced onion

Recipe:
1. Mix all the ingredients in your Instant Pot.
2. Cook on Stew for 10 minutes.
3. Release the pressure naturally.

DUCK STEW

Prep time: 15 minutes   **Setting:** Stew
Cooking time: 10 minutes   **Serves:** 2
Nutrition per serving:
Calories: 360   Carbs: 8   Sugar: 2

Fat: 20   Protein: 45   GL: 6

Ingredients:

- 1lb cooked diced duck breast
- 1lb chopped vegetables
- 1 cup chicken broth
- 1 cup whole button mushrooms
- 1tbsp mixed herbs

Recipe:

1. Mix all the ingredients in your Instant Pot.
2. Cook on Stew for 10 minutes.
3. Release the pressure naturally.

BEANSPROUT SOUP

Prep time: 15 minutes
Cooking time: 10 minutes
Setting: Stew
Serves: 2

Nutrition per serving:

Calories: 100	Sugar: 1	Protein: 4
Carbs: 4	Fat: 10	GL: 2

Ingredients:

- 1lb beansprouts
- 1lb chopped vegetables
- 1 cup low sodium broth
- 1tbsp mixed herbs
- 1 minced onion

Recipe:

1. Mix all the ingredients in your Instant Pot.
2. Cook on Stew for 10 minutes.
3. Release the pressure naturally.

HAM HOCK SOUP

Prep time: 15 minutes
Cooking time: 10 minutes
Setting: Stew
Serves: 2

Nutrition per serving:

Calories: 200	Carbs: 10	Sugar: 3

Fat: 15   Protein: 25   GL: 5

Ingredients:

- 1lb ham hock on the bone
- 1lb green peas
- 1 cup vegetable broth
- 1 cup shredded cabbage and onion
- 1tbsp mixed herbs

Recipe:

1. Mix all the ingredients in your Instant Pot.
2. Cook on Stew for 10 minutes.
3. Release the pressure naturally.

WHITE FISH AND TOMATO STEW

Cooking Time: 5 Minutes   Yield: 3 Servings

Main Ingredient

½ cup tomato sauce
1 teaspoon of garlic
2 tablespoons of olive oil
1 teaspoon oregano leaves

2 pounds f whitefish steaks, sliced
Salt and black pepper, to taste
2 white onions, chopped

Directions

1. Turn on sauté mode of the instant pot. Pour olive oil to the instant pot.
2. Add onions and garlic and cook until aroma comes. Then add oregano.
3. Sprinkle salt and black pepper on top. Cook for 1 minute. Then add fish and sear from both sides. Add tomato sauce and lock the lid. Set timer to 2 minutes.
4. Open timer beeps, release the steam quickly. Open the pot and serve hot.

EGGPLANT AND GREEK YOGURT STEW

Cooking Time: 10 Minutes   Yield: 8 Servings

Ingredients

6 large eggplants
1/3 cup finely chopped tomato
½ cup chopped onion

1/3 cup coconut amino
1-1/2 cups of Greek yogurt
6 tablespoons olive oil

Salt and black pepper, to taste

Directions

1. Heat oil in a skillet and add onions. Cook until translucent.
2. Add chopped tomatoes, coconut amino and cook for one minute.
3. Then add eggplants and salt and black pepper. Cook for 2 minutes.
4. Add Greek yogurt and lock the lid. Set timer for 4 minutes at high.
5. Release the steam quickly once timer beeps.
6. Open the pot and stir the ingredients, then serve.

SALMON AND BROCCOLI IN INSTANT POT

Cooking Time: 3 Minutes   **Yield:** 2-4 Servings

Ingredients

4 tablespoons of olive oil
Salt and black pepper, to taste
1.5 pounds of salmon fillets
1 teaspoon of spice mix, personal preference

1 lime, thinly sliced
2 small heads of broccoli, cut into large pieces

Directions

1. Grease the bottom of the instant pot with oil spray. Add broccoli to the instant pot and pour ¼ cup of water. Sprinkle salt, and pepper over the broccoli.
2. Place trivet on top of broccoli. Make a sling of aluminum foil on top of the trivet.
3. Layer lime and fish on the aluminum covered trivet.
4. Make sure fillets not lay over each other. Sprinkle spice mix over fillets.
5. Place a small piece of aluminum foil over the fish.
6. Lock the instant pot and set the timer to 3 minutes at high pressure.
7. Once timer beeps, quick release the steam.
8. Use a spatula to transfer the fish fillets to serving plates.
9. Carefully remove the broccoli from the bottom. Serve and enjoy.

PORK TENDERLOIN

Cooking Time: 27 Minutes   **Yield:** 2 Servings

Ingredients

3 tablespoons of olive oil

1 pound of pork tenderloin

2 cherries, peeled

1 onion, peeled

½ cup white vinegar

½ cup of stevia

Salt and black pepper, to taste

Directions

1. Turn on sauté mode of instant pot. Add olive oil to the pot.
2. Sear the pork tenderloin in the instant pot, for 2 minutes each side.
3. Transfer it onto the plate. Then add cherries, onion and vinegar.
4. Scrap the bottom of the instant pot.
5. Reduce the sauce to half and then add salt and black pepper.
6. Now, rub the pork tenderloin with stevia and place back in the instant pot.
7. Cover the pot with lid and set the timer to 22 minutes at high pressure.
8. Once timer beeps, release the steam naturally for 10 minutes. Once done serve and enjoy.

INSTANT POT SALMON WITH CHILI-LIME SAUCE

Cooking Time: 4 Minutes   **Yield: 1 Serving**

Ingredients

For Steaming Salmon

10 ounces of salmon fillets   Salt and black pepper

Ingredients for the Chili-Lime Sauce

1 lime juice

1 jalapeno, chopped

1 tablespoon of stevia

½ teaspoon of red chili

4 tablespoons of olive oil

Directions

1. Combine all the sauce ingredients in a bowl and set-asides for further use.
2. Now pour water about a cup in instant pot. Adjust steaming rack on top.
3. Season the salmon with salt and black pepper. Make a sling of aluminum foil on top of the trivet. Place salmon on a trivet and lock the lid.

4. Cook on high for 4 minutes. Once timer beeps, quick release the steam.
5. Open the instant Pot and transfer the salmon to a serving plate.
6. Serve with chili-lime sauce. Enjoy.

CHICKEN BREAST IN INSTANT POT

Cooking Time: 12 Minutes　　　　　　Yield:　1 Serving
Ingredients

2 chicken breasts

Salt and pepper

1 teaspoon of garlic powder

1 teaspoon of onion powder

Directions
1. Pour 2 cups of water in the instant pot. Adjust trivet on top.
2. Season the chicken breast with salt, pepper, garlic powder, and onion powder.
3. Place chicken on a trivet. Close the lid of the instant pot. Pressure cooks at high for 12 minutes. Then quickly release the steam. Unlock the instant pot.
4. Transfer chicken breast on cutting board and let it sit for 5 minutes.
5. Shred the chicken using the fork. Enjoy.

THAI CURRY ZUCCHINI INSTANT POT STEW

Cooking Time: 10 Minutes　　　　　　Yield:　2 Servings
Ingredients

4 cups of zucchini, peeled and chopped

½ teaspoon of curry paste, Thai

1 teaspoon of stevia

¼ cup of coconut milk

½ cup chicken broth

Directions
1. Dump all the ingredients in instant pot. Set the timer to 10 minutes after locking the lid.
2. Once timer beeps, quick release the steam. Stir the mixture and serve the stew.

COCONUT CONFECTION

Cooking Time: 12 Minutes   Yield: 4 Servings

Ingredients

2 cups of shredded coconut, dry   ½ cup of roasted almonds
2 cups of coconut milk   2 teaspoons of coconut oil
1/3 cup of stevia   1 tablespoon of Cardamom

Directions

1. Turn on the instant pot sauté mode and add shredded coconut, cardamom.
2. Mix and add half of the oil. Stir it well and cook for 1 minute. Pour in the coconut milk.
3. Set timer for 10 minutes at low pressure. Once timer beeps, quick release the steam.
4. Open the lid and add roasted almonds. Stir and add stevia. Mix the ingredient well and turn on sauté mode. Add remaining oil and stir for 2 minutes. Then serve.

BLACKBERRY CHEESECAKE IN AN INSTANT POT

Cooking Time: 30 Minutes   Yield: 4 Servings

Ingredients

16 ounces of coconut milk   1 teaspoon of cardamom
1 cup Greek yogurt   powder
1 cup blackberries puree   ½ cup Mix nuts, for garnish

Directions

1. Combine coconut milk, cardamom powder, mix nuts, blackberries, and yogurt in a bowl.
2. Pour the mixture into a greased pan that fits inside the pot.
3. Pour 2 cups of water in the pot. Set the trivet inside the instant pot.
4. Place grease pan on top of the trivet.
5. Lock the lid and set the timer to 30 minutes at high pressure.
6. Once the timer beeps naturally release steam for 20 minutes.
7. If the cake is not set, pressure cook for 3 more minutes.
8. Once the cake is set and not wiggly, it's done. Serve after chilling for 4 hours.

INSTANT POT VANILLA LAVA CAKE

Cooking Time: 101 Minutes   **Yield: 2 Servings**

Ingredients

2 large eggs

4 tablespoons of almond flour

13 ounces of coconut milk

3 tablespoons of stevia

½ teaspoon of Baking soda, dissolved

Directions

1. Pour coconut milk in a small stainless steel bowl.
2. Combine baking soda in water about 6 tablespoons and then add to the coconut milk.
3. Pour 2 cups of water in the instant pot. Place the stainless steel bowl in the water.
4. Lock the id and let it pressure cook for 90 minutes at high.
5. Quick release the steam after 90 minutes and open the pot.
6. If the desired color is not obtained, then re-cook for 30 more minutes at high pressure.
7. Once the desired color is obtained, transfer the stainless steel bowl to kitchen rack.
8. Now spray the ramekins with oil spray. Beat eggs until fluffy and then add prepared caramel. Then add almond flour and stevia. Mix it well.
9. Pour the mixture into greased ramekin cup. Now drain out the baking soda water from the pot. Add 2 cups of water to the instant pot and set trivet on top.
10. Place the ramekin on top of the trivet. Set timer for 11 minutes at high.
11. Once timer beeps, do a quick release. Remove cakes from the instant pot. Serve.

INSTANT POT CHIPOTLE BRISKET

Cooking Time: 70 Minutes   **Yield: 3 Servings**

Ingredients

3 pounds beef brisket

1 tablespoon bacon fat/lard

3 tablespoons chipotle seasoning

1 cup of water

Salt, to taste

1/3 cup cilantro, chopped and for garnish

Directions

1. Cut the beef brisket in equal parts. Turn on sauté mode of the instant pot and add bacon fat. Season the meat with chipotle powder and salt.
2. Melt the bacon fat and then sear the meat in the instant pot for 4 minutes per side.
3. Do in batches.
4. Once the beef is browned, add all meat pieces back to the instant pot along with water.
5. Close the instant pot lid. Set the timer to 70 minutes at high pressure.
6. Use meat. Stew button function. Once timer beeps, release the steam naturally for 15 minutes. Slice the beef and garnish with cilantro.

INSTANT POT CRACK CHICKEN RECIPE WITH CHEESE

Cooking Time: Minutes   **Yield: 6 Servings**

Ingredients

3 pounds of chicken breasts

10 ounces of cheddar cheese

1 cup of water

3 tablespoons of hot sauce

10 ounces of cream cheese

Salt and black pepper, to taste

Directions

1. Add water and chicken in the instant pot. Lock the Lid and pressure cooking at high for 10 minutes. Release steam naturally for 10 minutes.
2. Open the pot and then remove the chicken into the plate.
3. Discard the juice from the bottom of the instant pot. Add chicken back to the instant pot.
4. Shred the chicken into pieces with a fork inside the pot.
5. Add cream cheese, shredded cheddar cheese, and hot sauce to the pot.
6. Set the setting on keeps warm. Stir the ingredients and waits until the cheese melts.
7. Season it with salt and pepper. Serve.

Light Meals And Appetizers

Depending on how your day is going, you might need something small to eat instead of your usual meal, or you might need an appetizer to help make sure you are eating enough. All these recipes are under 150 calories, so they are perfect for this.

EGG FRIED VEG

Prep time: 10 minutes   **Setting:** Steam
Cooking time: 7 minutes   **Serves:** 2
Nutrition per serving:

Calories: 100	Sugar: 1	Protein: 15
Carbs: 7	Fat: 1	GL: 2

Ingredients:
- 4oz egg whites
- 1 cup mixed vegetables
- 2tbsp milk
- zero calorie spray
- herb and spice mix

Recipe:
1. Spray a heat-proof bowl that fits in your Instant Pot with nonstick spray.
2. Whisk together the eggs, milk, and seasoning.
3. Pour into the bowl. Add the vegetables.
4. Place the bowl in your steamer basket.
5. Pour 1 cup of water into your Instant Pot.
6. Lower the basket into your Instant Pot.
7. Seal and cook on low pressure for 7 minutes.
8. Depressurize quickly.
9. Stir well and allow to rest, it will finish cooking in its own heat.

BONE BROTH

Prep time: 10 minutes
Cooking time: 60 minutes
Nutrition per serving:

Setting: Manual
Serves: 2

Calories: 38
Carbs: 2

Sugar: 0
Fat: 2

Protein: 3
GL: 1

Ingredients:
- 1 chicken carcass and dripping OR 1 large marrow bone
- 1 chopped onion
- 1 stalk chopped celery
- 1 tbsp minced garlic
- 1 tbsp bouillon powder

Recipe:
1. Place the chicken, onion, and celery in your Instant Pot.
2. Cover with 2 cups of water.
3. Seal and cook on Manual, high pressure, for 60 minutes.
4. Release the pressure naturally.
5. Strain the solids out.
6. Add the garlic and bouillon.

CAULIFLOWER AND CELERIAC SOUP

Prep time: 15 minutes
Cooking time: 10 minutes
Nutrition per serving:

Setting: Stew.
Serves: 2

Calories: 125
Carbs: 16

Sugar: 2
Fat: 2

Protein: 6
GL: 3

Ingredients:
- 0.5lb cauliflower, chopped
- 4oz celeriac, chopped
- 1 chopped onion
- 2 cups vegetable stock
- salt and pepper

Recipe:
1. Mix all the ingredients in your Instant Pot.
2. Cook on Stew for 10 minutes.

3. Depressurize naturally and blend.

MUSHROOM AND EGGS

Prep time: 10 minutes   **Setting:** Steam
Cooking time: 7 minutes   **Serves:** 2
Nutrition per serving:

Calories: 80	Sugar: 0	Protein: 15
Carbs: 2	Fat: 1	GL: 2

Ingredients:
- 4oz egg whites
- 1 cup chopped brown mushrooms
- 2tbsp milk
- zero calorie spray
- 1tsp mustard

Recipe:
1. Spray a heat-proof bowl that fits in your Instant Pot with nonstick spray.
2. Whisk together the eggs, milk, and seasoning.
3. Pour into the bowl. Add the mushroom.
4. Place the bowl in your steamer basket.
5. Pour 1 cup of water into your Instant Pot.
6. Lower the basket into your Instant Pot.
7. Seal and cook on low pressure for 7 minutes. Depressurize quickly.
8. Stir well and allow to rest, it will finish cooking in its own heat.

CARROT AND CILANTRO SOUP

Prep time: 15 minutes   **Setting:** Stew.
Cooking time: 10 minutes   **Serves:** 2
Nutrition per serving:

Calories: 90	Sugar: 2	Protein: 3
Carbs: 9	Fat: 2	GL: 2

Ingredients:
- 2 cups chopped carrot
- 2 chopped onions

- 2 cups vegetable stock
- 1 cup chopped cilantro

Recipe:
1. Mix all the ingredients in your Instant Pot.
2. Cook on Stew for 10 minutes.
3. Depressurize naturally and blend.

RATATOUILLE

Prep time: 15 minutes

Cooking time: 10 minutes

Setting: Stew.

Serves: 2

Nutrition per serving:

Calories: 100	Sugar: 4	Protein: 3
Carbs: 7	Fat: 2	GL: 1

Ingredients:
- 2 chopped beef tomatoes
- 1 chopped eggplant
- 1 chopped zucchini
- 1 chopped onion
- 2 cups vegetable stock

Recipe:
1. Mix all the ingredients in your Instant Pot.
2. Cook on Stew for 10 minutes.
3. Depressurize naturally.

TOMATO EGGS

Prep time: 10 minutes

Cooking time: 7 minutes

Setting: Steam

Serves: 2

Nutrition per serving:

Calories: 100	Sugar: 4	Protein: 15
Carbs: 6	Fat: 1	GL: 3

Ingredients:
- 4oz egg whites
- 2tbsp milk
- zero calorie spray

- 0.5 cup chopped cherry tomatoes
- 0.5 cup chopped bell peppers, mixed colors

Recipe:
1. Spray a heat-proof bowl that fits in your Instant Pot with nonstick spray.
2. Whisk together the eggs, milk, and add a pinch of salt.
3. Pour into the bowl. Add the vegetables.
4. Place the bowl in your steamer basket.
5. Pour 1 cup of water into your Instant Pot.
6. Lower the basket into your Instant Pot.
7. Seal and cook on low pressure for 7 minutes. Depressurize quickly.
8. Stir well and allow to rest, it will finish cooking in its own heat.

HERB CRUSTED CHICKEN

Prep time: 10 minutes
Cooking time: 10 minutes
Setting: Saute
Serves: 2
Nutrition per serving:

Calories: 63	Sugar: 2	Protein: 7
Carbs: 3	Fat: 3	GL: 1

Ingredients:
- 2oz chopped chicken breast
- 1 chopped sweet pepper
- 1 cup chopped sugar snap peas
- 1/4 cup chopped fresh herbs
- 2tbsp olive oil

Recipe:
1. Pat the chicken and vegetables dry and roll 1tbsp of the oil.
2. Roll in the herbs.
3. Put the other 1tbsp of oil into the Instant Pot.
4. Cook on Saute for 10 minutes.
5. Ensure the chicken is cooked through before serving.

CARROT HUMMUS

Prep time: 15 minutes
Cooking time: 10 minutes
Nutrition per serving:

Setting: Stew
Serves: 2

Calories: 58
Carbs: 8

Sugar: 2
Fat: 2

Protein: 2
GL: 2

Ingredients:
- 1 small chopped carrot
- 2oz cooked chickpeas
- 1tsp lemon juice
- 1tsp tahini
- 1tsp fresh parsley

Recipe:
1. Place the carrot and chickpeas in your Instant Pot.
2. Add a cup of water, seal.
3. Cook for 10 minutes on Stew.
4. Depressurize naturally.
5. Blend with the remaining ingredients.

MUSHROOM TOFU SCRAMBLE

Prep time: 15 minutes
Cooking time: 7 minutes
Nutrition per serving:

Setting: Steam
Serves: 2

Calories: 120
Carbs: 3

Sugar: 1
Fat: 3

Protein: 18
GL: 1

Ingredients:
- 1 cup firm tofu
- 1 cup chopped mixed mushrooms
- 3tbsp mushroom soup
- 1tsp mixed herbs
- pinch of salt

Recipe:
1. Spray a heat-proof bowl that fits in your Instant Pot with nonstick spray.
2. Chop the tofu finely.

3. Mix with the other ingredients. Pour into the bowl.
4. Place the bowl in your steamer basket.
5. Pour 1 cup of water into your Instant Pot. Lower the basket into your Instant Pot.
6. Seal and cook on low pressure for 7 minutes. Depressurize quickly.
7. Stir well and allow to rest, it will finish cooking in its own heat.

LENTIL SOUP

Prep time: 10 minutes
Cooking time: 20 minutes
Setting: Beans
Serves: 2
Nutrition per serving:

| Calories: 70 | Sugar: 4 | Protein: 7 |
| Carbs: 18 | Fat: 0 | GL: 3 |

Ingredients:
- 3oz dry lentils
- 1/4 cup sliced leek
- 1 small chopped carrot
- 1 chopped celery stalk
- 1/4 cup tomato sauce

Recipe:
1. Place all the ingredients in your Instant Pot.
2. Seal and cook on Beans for 20 minutes.
3. Depressurize naturally.

STUFFED MUSHROOMS

Prep time: 15 minutes
Cooking time: 5 minutes
Setting: Steam
Serves: 2
Nutrition per serving:

| Calories: 100 | Sugar: 1 | Protein: 2 |
| Carbs: 2 | Fat: 1 | GL: 1 |

Ingredients:
- 10 1-2" mushrooms, stalks removed
- 0.5 cup minced broccoli
- 0.5 minced onion
- 1 clove minced garlic
- salt and pepper

Recipe:

1. Rinse the mushrooms.
2. Mix the other ingredients together and stuff them into the mushrooms.
3. Place the mushrooms carefully in your Instant Pot steamer basket.
4. Pour a cup of water into the Instant Pot and insert the steamer basket.
5. Cook on Steam for 5 minutes.
6. Depressurize naturally and serve right away.

EGGPLANT TOFU SCRAMBLE

Prep time: 15 minutes   **Setting:** Steam
Cooking time: 7 minutes   **Serves:** 2
Nutrition per serving:

Calories: 130	Sugar: 1	Protein: 19
Carbs: 5	Fat: 3	GL: 1

Ingredients:

- 1 cup firm tofu
- 1 cup roughly chopped eggplant
- 3tbsp low calorie stock
- 1tsp mustard
- pinch of salt

Recipe:

1. Spray a heat-proof bowl that fits in your Instant Pot with nonstick spray.
2. Chop the tofu finely. Mix with the other ingredients. Pour into the bowl.
3. Place the bowl in your steamer basket.
4. Pour 1 cup of water into your Instant Pot. Lower the basket into your Instant Pot.
5. Seal and cook on low pressure for 7 minutes. Depressurize quickly.
6. Stir well and allow to rest, it will finish cooking in its own heat.

SPINACH DIP

Prep time: 5 minutes   **Cooking time:** 2 minutes

Setting: Stew   **Serves:** 2

Nutrition per serving:

Calories: 112   Sugar: 6   Protein: 6

Carbs: 8   Fat: 8   GL: 3

Ingredients:

- 1oz chopped spinach
- 1oz low fat plain yogurt
- 1tbsp peanut butter
- 1tsp honey
- 1/4tsp chili pepper

Recipe:

1. Place the spinach, yogurt, and peanut butter in a heat-proof bowl.
2. Pour a cup of water into the Instant Pot.
3. Place the bowl in the steamer basket and the basket in the Instant Pot.
4. Cook on Stew, low pressure for 2 minutes.
5. Release the pressure quickly.
6. Stir well and add the honey and chili.

CABBAGE SOUP

Prep time: 15 minutes   **Setting:** Stew.

Cooking time: 10 minutes   **Serves:** 2

Nutrition per serving:

Calories: 12   Sugar: 0   Protein: 1

Carbs: 2   Fat: 0   GL: 1

Ingredients:

- 2 cups finely shredded savoy cabbage
- 1 cup finely shredded red cabbage
- 1 cup chopped scallions
- 2 cups vegetable stock
- salt and pepper

Recipe:

1. Mix all the ingredients in your Instant Pot.
2. Cook on Stew for 10 minutes.
3. Depressurize naturally and blend.

Side Dishes

So many side dishes are either carbs or salads. But when your main meal is full of vegetables already and carbs are off the menu for a while, you need to get creative with your side dishes to keep things fresh.

LOW FAT ROASTIES

Prep time: 10 minutes.
Cooking time: 25 minutes.

Setting: Saute.
Serves: 2

Nutrition per serving:

Calories: 201   Sugar: 1   Protein: 5
Carbs: 35   Fat: 6   GL: 26

Ingredients:

- 1lb roasting potatoes
- 1 garlic clove
- 1 cup vegetable stock
- 2tbsp olive oil

Recipe:

1. Put the potatoes in the steamer basket and add the stock into the Instant Pot.
2. Steam the potatoes in your Instant Pot for 15 minutes.
3. Depressurize and pour away the remaining stock.
4. Set to saute and add the oil, garlic, and potatoes. Cook until brown.

CHILI GREENS

Prep time: 10 minutes
Cooking time: 10 minutes

Setting: Stew
Serves: 2

Nutrition per serving:

Calories: 60   Sugar: 1   Protein: 2
Carbs: 12   Fat: 0   GL: 4

Ingredients:

- 2 cups mixed cabbage, shredded
- 1 cup trimmed green beans
- 3 stalks chopped scallions

- 2tbsp chili paste
- salt and pepper to taste

Recipe:
1. Mix the ingredients in the Instant Pot.
2. Seal and cook on Stew for 10 minutes. Depressurize naturally.

CARAMELIZED CARROT AND ONION

Prep time: 10
Cooking time: 15

Setting: Saute.
Serves: 2

Nutrition per serving:

Calories: 129	Sugar: 13	Protein: 2
Carbs: 15	Fat: 7	GL: 16

Ingredients:
- 0.5lb carrot, peeled and chopped into fingers
- 2 red onions, peeled and quartered
- 3tbsp red wine
- 2tbsp butter
- 2tbsp herbs
- 1tbsp olive oil
- 1tbsp honey
- 1tbsp balsamic vinegar

Recipe:
1. Blanch the carrots in boiling water for 3 minutes.
2. Drain them, put them in your Instant Pot with butter and oil, and fry carrots, onions, and herbs on Saute until brown.
3. Add the honey, wine, and balsamic.
4. Saute until thick and syrupy.

LOWER CARB HUMMUS

Prep time: 30 minutes
Cooking time: 60 minutes

Setting: Beans.
Serves: 2

Nutrition per serving:

Calories: 135	Sugar: 2	Protein: 13
Carbs: 18	Fat: 3	GL: 6

Ingredients:
- 0.5 cup dry chickpeas
- 1 cup vegetable stock

- 1 cup pumpkin puree
- 2tbsp smoked paprika
- salt and pepper to taste

Recipe:
1. Soak the chickpeas overnight.
2. Place the chickpeas and stock in the Instant Pot.
3. Cook on Beans 60 minutes.
4. Depressurize naturally.
5. Blend the chickpeas with the remaining ingredients.

HUMMUS DAHL

Prep time: 30 minutes
Cooking time: 60 minutes
Setting: Beans.
Serves: 2
Nutrition per serving:

Calories: 135	Sugar: 1	Protein: 15
Carbs: 14	Fat: 10	GL: 5

Ingredients:
- 0.5 cup dry lentils
- 0.5 cup pumpkin puree
- 1 cup vegetable stock
- 2tbsp light tahini

Recipe:
1. Soak the lentils overnight.
2. Place the lentils and stock in the Instant Pot.
3. Cook on Beans 60 minutes.
4. Depressurize naturally.
5. Blend the lentils with the remaining ingredients.

CARROT AND SWEDE

Prep time: 10 minutes
Cooking time: 15 minutes
Setting: Stew.
Serves: 2
Nutrition per serving:

Calories: 60	Sugar: 1	Protein: 2
Carbs: 10	Fat: 1	GL: 1

Ingredients:
- 1 cup chopped carrots
- 1 cup chopped swede
- 1 cup vegetable broth
- 2tbsp minced garlic

Recipe:
1. Place the ingredients in your Instant Pot.
2. Seal and cook on Stew 15 minutes.
3. Strain any excess broth.
4. Mash the carrots and swede until the texture is as desired.

ROASTED PARSNIPS

Prep time: 10 minutes.
Cooking time: 25 minutes.
Setting: Saute.
Serves: 2
Nutrition per serving:

| Calories: 130 | Sugar: 0 | Protein: 4 |
| Carbs: 14 | Fat: 6 | GL: 16 |

Ingredients:
- 1lb parsnips
- 1 cup vegetable stock
- 2tbsp herbs
- 2tbsp olive oil

Recipe:
1. Put the parsnips in the steamer basket and add the stock into the Instant Pot.
2. Steam the parsnips in your Instant Pot for 15 minutes.
3. Depressurize and pour away the remaining stock.
4. Set to saute and add the oil, herbs and parsnips.
5. Cook until golden and crisp.

HONEY PARSNIPS

Prep time: 10
Cooking time: 15
Setting: Saute.
Serves: 2
Nutrition per serving:

| Calories: 135 | Carbs: 17 | Sugar: 13 |

Fat: 7   Protein: 2   GL: 17

Ingredients:

- 1lb parsnips, peeled and chopped into fingers
- 3tbsp white or rose wine
- 3tbsp butter
- 2tbsp rosemary
- 1tbsp honey
- 1tbsp balsamic vinegar

Recipe:

1. Place the parsnips in your Instant Pot with butter and parsnips and rosemary, put on Saute until brown.
2. Add the honey, wine, and balsamic.
3. Saute until thick and syrupy.

ROSEMARY POTATOES

Prep time: 10 minutes.   **Setting:** Saute.
Cooking time: 25 minutes.   **Serves:** 2
Nutrition per serving:

Calories: 195   Sugar: 1   Protein: 5
Carbs: 31   Fat: 6   GL: 25

Ingredients:

- 1lb red potatoes
- 1 cup vegetable stock
- 2tbsp olive oil
- 2tbsp rosemary sprigs

Recipe:

1. Put the potatoes in the steamer basket and add the stock into the Instant Pot.
2. Steam the potatoes in your Instant Pot for 15 minutes.
3. Depressurize and pour away the remaining stock.
4. Set to saute and add the oil, rosemary, and potatoes.
5. Cook until brown.

MASHED PUMPKIN

Prep time: 10
Cooking time: 15
Nutrition per serving:

Setting: Stew.
Serves: 2

| Calories: 12 | Sugar: 1 | Protein: 0 |
| Carbs: 3 | Fat: 0 | GL: 1 |

Ingredients:
- 2 cups chopped pumpkin
- 0.5 cup water
- 2tbsp powdered sugar-free sweetener of choice
- 1tbsp cinnamon

Recipe:
1. Place the pumpkin and water in your Instant Pot.
2. Seal and cook on Stew 15 minutes.
3. Remove and mash with the sweetener and cinnamon.

Meat Dishes

Meat is a huge staple of many diabetics' diets. This is because a lean meat adds much needed protein without adding any carbohydrate or much fat, protecting your pancreas and gallbladder. In this section we shall see how red meats can be made into simple five ingredient meals to suit a diabetic diet. Side of fries not needed!

TRADITIONAL BEEF STEW

Prep time: 15 minutes
Cooking time: 35 minutes
Nutrition per serving:

Setting: Stew
Serves: 2

Calories: 300	Sugar: 1	Protein: 43
Carbs: 6	Fat: 9	GL: 2

Ingredients:
- 1lb diced stewing steak
- 1lb chopped vegetables
- 1 cup low sodium beef broth
- 1tbsp black pepper

Recipe:
1. Mix all the ingredients in your Instant Pot.
2. Cook on Stew for 35 minutes. Release the pressure naturally.

FABADA

Prep time: 15 minutes
Cooking time: 5 minutes
Nutrition per serving:

Setting: Stew
Serves: 2

Calories: 300	Sugar: 2	Protein: 35
Carbs: 20	Fat: 15	GL: 9

Ingredients:
- 0.5lb cubed ham
- 0.5lb black pudding
- 1lb cooked beans
- 1 cup low sodium broth

- 1tbsp spicy seasoning

Recipe:
1. Mix all the ingredients in your Instant Pot.
2. Cook on Stew for 5 minutes. Release the pressure naturally.

STEAK AND KIDNEY STEW

Prep time: 15 minutes
Cooking time: 35 minutes
Nutrition per serving:

Setting: Stew
Serves: 2

Calories: 380   Sugar: 3   Protein: 48
Carbs: 10   Fat: 12   GL: 4

Ingredients:
- 1lb diced stewing steak
- 0.5lb diced kidneys
- 1lb chopped vegetables
- 1 cup low sodium beef broth
- 0.5 cup low carb beer

Recipe:
1. Mix all the ingredients in your Instant Pot.
2. Cook on Stew for 35 minutes.
3. Release the pressure naturally.

SLOW COOKED LAMB

Prep time: 15 minutes
Cooking time: 35 minutes
Nutrition per serving:

Setting: Stew
Serves: 2

Calories: 400   Sugar: 4   Protein: 37
Carbs: 14   Fat: 20   GL: 6

Ingredients:
- 1lb diced lean lamb
- 1 quartered onion
- 2 chopped carrots
- 1 cup low sodium broth
- 0.5 cup mint sauce

Recipe:

1. Place the lamb in your Instant Pot.
2. Place the onion and carrots around it.
3. Pour the sauce and broth over it.
4. Cook on Stew for 35 minutes.
5. Release the pressure naturally.

HONEY MUSTARD PORK

Prep time: 15 minutes

Cooking time: 60 minutes

Setting: Stew

Serves: 2

Nutrition per serving:

Calories: 290	Sugar: 8	Protein: 39
Carbs: 9	Fat: 17	GL: 4

Ingredients:

- 1.5lb rolled, trimmed pork joint
- 1 cup honey mustard sauce, low carb
- salt and pepper

Recipe:

1. Mix all the ingredients in your Instant Pot.
2. Cook on Stew for 60 minutes.
3. Release the pressure naturally.

SHREDDED BEEF

Prep time: 15 minutes

Cooking time: 35 minutes

Setting: Stew

Serves: 2

Nutrition per serving:

Calories: 200	Sugar: 0	Protein: 48
Carbs: 2	Fat: 5	GL: 1

Ingredients:

- 1.5lb lean steak
- 1 cup low sodium gravy

- 2tbsp mixed spices

Recipe:
1. Mix all the ingredients in your Instant Pot.
2. Cook on Stew for 35 minutes.
3. Release the pressure naturally.
4. Shred the beef.

ITALIAN SAUSAGE CASSEROLE

Prep time: 15 minutes
Cooking time: 5 minutes

Setting: Stew
Serves: 2

Nutrition per serving:

Calories: 320	Sugar: 2	Protein: 41
Carbs: 8	Fat: 18	GL: 4

Ingredients:
- 1lb chopped cooked sausages
- 1lb chopped Mediterranean vegetables
- 1 cup low sodium broth
- 1tbsp mixed herbs

Recipe:
1. Mix all the ingredients in your Instant Pot.
2. Cook on Stew for 5 minutes.
3. Release the pressure naturally.

ROAST BEEF

Prep time: 15 minutes
Cooking time: 60 minutes

Setting: Stew
Serves: 2

Nutrition per serving:

Calories: 275	Sugar: 0	Protein: 49
Carbs: 5	Fat: 7	GL: 2

Ingredients:
- 1lb trimmed, tied beef joint
- 1lb cubed winter vegetables
- 1 cup low sodium beef broth
- 1 cup gravy

Recipe:
1. Mix the broth and gravy.
2. Place the beef in your Instant Pot.
3. Pour the broth and gravy on top.
4. Cook on Stew for 60 minutes.
5. Release the pressure naturally.

PULLED PORK

Prep time: 15 minutes
Cooking time: 35 minutes
Nutrition per serving:

Setting: Stew
Serves: 2

Calories: 340	Sugar: 1	Protein: 45
Carbs: 4	Fat: 22	GL: 1

Ingredients:
- 1.5lb cubed pork
- 1 cup low sodium beef broth
- 0.5 cup low carb BBQ sauce
- 1tbsp spices

Recipe:
1. Mix all the ingredients in your Instant Pot.
2. Cook on Stew for 35 minutes.
3. Release the pressure naturally.
4. Shred the pork.

CORNED BEEF STEW

Prep time: 15 minutes
Cooking time: 10 minutes
Nutrition per serving:

Setting: Stew
Serves: 2

Calories: 380	Sugar: 2	Protein: 38
Carbs: 9	Fat: 19	GL: 3

Ingredients:
- 1lb corned beef

- 1lb chopped winter vegetables
- 1 cup low sodium beef broth
- 1 cup green peas

Recipe:

1. Mix all the ingredients in your Instant Pot.
2. Cook on Stew for 10 minutes.
3. Release the pressure naturally.

LAMB AND MUSHROOM STEW

Prep time: 15 minutes
Cooking time: 35 minutes
Setting: Stew
Serves: 2

Nutrition per serving:

| Calories: 340 | Sugar: 0 | Protein: 45 |
| Carbs: 3 | Fat: 19 | GL: 1 |

Ingredients:

- 1lb diced lamb
- 1lb chopped vegetables
- 1 cup mushrooms
- 1 cup mushroom soup
- 1tbsp black pepper

Recipe:

1. Mix all the ingredients in your Instant Pot.
2. Cook on Stew for 35 minutes.
3. Release the pressure naturally.

OXTAIL SOUP

Prep time: 15 minutes
Cooking time: 35 minutes
Setting: Stew
Serves: 2

Nutrition per serving:

| Calories: 200 | Sugar: 0 | Protein: 37 |
| Carbs: 2 | Fat: 6 | GL: 1 |

Ingredients:

- 1lb of prepared ox tail

- 1lb chopped Mediterranean vegetables
- 1 cup low sodium beef broth

Recipe:
1. Mix all the ingredients in your Instant Pot.
2. Cook on Stew for 35 minutes.
3. Release the pressure naturally.

VEAL IN MILK

Prep time: 15 minutes
Cooking time: 35 minutes
Setting: Stew
Serves: 2
Nutrition per serving:

Calories: 270	Sugar: 0	Protein: 39
Carbs: 2	Fat: 16	GL: 1

Ingredients:
- 1lb veal steak
- 1lb chopped vegetables
- 2 cups whole milk
- 1tbsp black pepper seasoning mix

Recipe:
1. Mix all the ingredients in your Instant Pot.
2. Cook on Stew for 35 minutes.
3. Release the pressure naturally.

BEEF OFFAL STEW

Prep time: 15 minutes
Cooking time: 35 minutes
Setting: Stew
Serves: 2
Nutrition per serving:

Calories: 360	Sugar: 1	Protein: 48
Carbs: 8	Fat: 20	GL: 3

Ingredients:
- 0.5lb diced ox heart
- 0.5lb diced kidney

- 0.5lb cured, diced ox tongue
- 1lb chopped vegetables
- 1 cup low sodium beef broth

Recipe:

1. Mix all the ingredients in your Instant Pot.
2. Cook on Stew for 35 minutes.
3. Release the pressure naturally.

GOAT CURRY

Prep time: 15 minutes
Cooking time: 35 minutes
Setting: Stew
Serves: 2

Nutrition per serving:

| Calories: 390 | Sugar: 5 | Protein: 46 |
| Carbs: 12 | Fat: 19 | GL: 6 |

Ingredients:

- 1lb diced goat
- 1lb chopped vegetables
- 1 cup chopped tomato
- 1 cup low sodium beef broth
- 1tbsp curry paste

Recipe:

1. Mix all the ingredients in your Instant Pot.
2. Cook on Stew for 35 minutes.
3. Release the pressure naturally.

Poultry Dishes

If red meats are a diabetic staple, then poultry is an all-time favorite. Because chicken, duck, or turkey is much leaner than the average red meat, it does not affect your gallbladder the same way, which can help to protect your pancreas. And because these meats are so full of protein they make a wonderful, filling base for a diabetic meal.

TURKEY AND PARSNIPS CURRY

Prep time: 15 minutes
Cooking time: 20 minutes
Setting: Stew.
Serves: 2
Nutrition per serving:

Calories: 400	Sugar: 16	Protein: 43
Carbs: 27	Fat: 15	GL: 21

Ingredients:
- 0.5lb parsnip
- 0.5lb chopped cooked turkey
- 1 thinly sliced onion
- 1 cup curry sauce
- 1tbsp oil or ghee

Recipe:
1. Set the Instant Pot to saute and add the onion and oil.
2. When the onion is soft, add the remaining ingredients and seal.
3. Cook on Stew for 20 minutes.
4. Release the pressure naturally.
5.

TURKEY DINNER CASSEROLE

Prep time: 15 minutes
Cooking time: 10 minutes
Setting: Stew
Serves: 2
Nutrition per serving:

Calories: 400	Sugar: 18	Protein: 39
Carbs: 34	Fat: 13	GL: 20

Ingredients:
- 1lb cooked shredded turkey
- 1lb chopped vegetables
- 1 cup low sugar honey mustard sauce
- 1tbsp mixed herbs

- 1 minced onion

Recipe:
1. Mix all the ingredients in your Instant Pot.
2. Cook on Stew for 10 minutes. Release the pressure naturally.

PULLED CHICKEN

Prep time: 15 minutes
Cooking time: 35 minutes
Nutrition per serving:

Setting: Stew
Serves: 2

Calories: 290	Sugar: 4	Protein: 45
Carbs: 7	Fat: 7	GL: 4

Ingredients:
- 1.5lb chicken breast
- 2 shredded onions
- 1 cup low sodium broth
- 1 cup BBQ sauce

Recipe:
1. Mix all the ingredients in your Instant Pot.
2. Cook on Stew for 35 minutes.
3. Release the pressure naturally.
4. Shred the chicken.

HALF ROAST CHICKEN

Prep time: 15 minutes
Cooking time: 35 minutes
Nutrition per serving:

Setting: Stew
Serves: 2

Calories: 300	Sugar: 1	Protein: 43
Carbs: 6	Fat: 9	GL: 2

Ingredients:
- half a chicken
- 2tbsp mixed herbs
- 2tbsp rub
- 1 cup low sodium broth

Recipe:

1. Mix all the herbs, rub, and a little broth and rub it into the chicken.
2. Pour the broth in your Instant Pot and lower the chicken, bones down.
3. Cook on Stew for 35 minutes.
4. Release the pressure naturally.

TURKEY ZOODLES

Prep time: 15 minutes

Cooking time: 35 minutes

Nutrition per serving:

Calories: 250

Carbs: 4

Sugar: 0

Setting: Stew

Serves: 2

Fat: 7

Protein: 39

GL: 1

Ingredients:
- 1lb diced turkey
- 1lb spiralized zucchini
- 1 cup diced vegetables
- 1 cup low sodium chicken broth

Recipe:
1. Mix all the ingredients except the zucchini in your Instant Pot.
2. Cook on Stew for 35 minutes.
3. Release the pressure naturally.
4. Stir in the zucchini and allow to warm through before serving.

CHICKEN COCONUT CURRY

Prep time: 15 minutes

Cooking time: 20 minutes

Nutrition per serving:

Calories: 450

Carbs: 27

Sugar: 16

Fat: 25

Setting: Stew.

Serves: 2

Protein: 43

GL: 21

Ingredients:
- 0.5lb chopped cooked chicken breast
- 1 thinly sliced onion
- 1 cup coconut milk
- 3tbsp curry paste
- 1tbsp oil or ghee

Recipe:
1. Set the Instant Pot to saute and add the onion, oil, and curry paste.
2. When the onion is soft, add the remaining ingredients and seal.
3. Cook on Stew for 20 minutes.
4. Release the pressure naturally.

TURKEY MEATBALL STEW

Prep time: 15 minutes   **Setting:** Stew
Cooking time: 35 minutes   **Serves:** 2
Nutrition per serving:

Calories: 260	Sugar: 1	Protein: 38
Carbs: 6	Fat: 7	GL: 2

Ingredients:
- 1lb minced turkey
- 1lb chopped vegetables
- 1 cup chicken soup
- 3tbsp almond flour
- 2tbsp mixed seasoning

Recipe:
1. Roll the turkey into meatballs with the seasoning and almond flour.
2. Mix all the ingredients in your Instant Pot.
3. Cook on Stew for 35 minutes.
4. Release the pressure naturally.

DUCK AND BEAN STEW

Prep time: 15 minutes   **Setting:** Stew
Cooking time: 35 minutes   **Serves:** 2
Nutrition per serving:

Calories: 360	Sugar: 3	Protein: 39
Carbs: 16	Fat: 14	GL: 5

Ingredients:
- 1lb diced duck breast
- 1lb cooked black beans
- 1 cup low sodium vegetable broth

- 1 tbsp 5 spice seasoning

Recipe:
1. Mix all the ingredients in your Instant Pot.
2. Cook on Stew for 35 minutes.
3. Release the pressure naturally.

CHICKEN ZOODLE SOUP

Prep time: 15 minutes
Cooking time: 35 minutes
Setting: Stew
Serves: 2

Nutrition per serving:

Calories: 250	Sugar: 0	Protein: 40
Carbs: 5	Fat: 10	GL: 1

Ingredients:
- 1 lb chopped cooked chicken
- 1 lb spiralized zucchini
- 1 cup low sodium chicken soup
- 1 cup diced vegetables

Recipe:
1. Mix all the ingredients except the zucchini in your Instant Pot.
2. Cook on Stew for 35 minutes.
3. Release the pressure naturally.
4. Stir in the zucchini and allow to heat thoroughly.

TURKEY AND SPAGHETTI SQUASH

Prep time: 15 minutes
Cooking time: 35 minutes
Setting: Stew
Serves: 2

Nutrition per serving:

Calories: 260	Sugar: 0	Protein: 41
Carbs: 5	Fat: 5	GL: 1

Ingredients:
- 1 lb minced turkey
- 1 cup chicken broth
- 1 tbsp mixed Italian herbs
- 1/2 spaghetti squash, to fit the Instant Pot

Recipe:
1. Mix the herbs into the turkey.
2. Pack the turkey into the squash.
3. Pour the broth in your Instant Pot.
4. Put the squash into the Instant Pot.
5. Cook on Stew for 35 minutes.
6. Release the pressure naturally.
7. Shred the squash and mix the "spaghetti" with the turkey.

THAI GREEN TURKEY CURRY

Prep time: 15 minutes   **Setting:** Stew.
Cooking time: 20 minutes   **Serves:** 2
Nutrition per serving:
Calories: 350   Sugar: 5   Protein: 43
Carbs: 16   Fat: 15   GL: 12
Ingredients:
- 0.5lb chopped cooked turkey
- 0.5 cup minced scallions and greens
- 0.5 cup chopped tomato
- 3tbsp Thai green curry paste
- 1tbsp oil or ghee

Recipe:
1. Set the Instant Pot to saute and add the oil and curry paste.
2. When mixed, add the remaining ingredients and seal.
3. Cook on Stew for 20 minutes.
4. Release the pressure naturally.

DUCK IN ORANGE SAUCE

Prep time: 15 minutes   **Setting:** Stew
Cooking time: 35 minutes   **Serves:** 2
Nutrition per serving:
Calories: 315   Sugar: 7   Protein: 37
Carbs: 13   Fat: 16   GL: 4

Ingredients:
- 1lb diced duck breast
- 1lb stir fry vegetables
- 1 cup low sodium broth
- 1 cup orange juice
- 2tbsp marmalade

Recipe:
1. Mix all the ingredients in your Instant Pot.
2. Cook on Stew for 35 minutes.
3. Release the pressure naturally.

LEMON CILANTRO CHICKEN

Prep time: 15 minutes
Cooking time: 35 minutes
Setting: Stew
Serves: 2

Nutrition per serving:

Calories: 280	Sugar: 0	Protein: 45
Carbs: 4	Fat: 12	GL: 1

Ingredients:
- 1lb diced chicken breast
- 1lb chopped vegetables
- 1 cup chicken broth
- juice of half a lemon
- 2tbsp dry cilantro

Recipe:
1. Mix all the ingredients in your Instant Pot.
2. Cook on Stew for 35 minutes.
3. Release the pressure naturally.

CHICKEN LIVER CURRY

Prep time: 15 minutes
Cooking time: 35 minutes
Setting: Stew
Serves: 2

Nutrition per serving:

Calories: 350	Sugar: 2	Protein: 52
Carbs: 10	Fat: 17	GL: 4

Ingredients:

- 1lb diced chicken breast
- 0.5lb diced chicken liver
- 1lb chopped vegetables
- 1 cup broth
- 3tbsp curry paste

Recipe:

1. Mix all the ingredients in your Instant Pot.
2. Cook on Stew for 35 minutes.
3. Release the pressure naturally.

BALSAMIC TURKEY BREAST

Prep time: 15 minutes
Cooking time: 35 minutes
Setting: Stew
Serves: 2
Nutrition per serving:

Calories: 295	Sugar: 2	Protein: 46
Carbs: 5	Fat: 14	GL: 2

Ingredients:

- 1lb diced turkey breast
- 1lb chopped vegetables
- 1 cup chicken soup
- 2tbsp balsamic reduction

Recipe:

1. Mix all the ingredients in your Instant Pot.
2. Cook on Stew for 35 minutes.
3. Release the pressure naturally.

Seafood Dishes

Seafood is a perfect source of protein for a diabetic. It is low in carbs and very high in protein. It is also loaded with vitamins and minerals that you do not find in most land meats, such as those all important ones: Vitamin D and chromium. If you need to eat less fat, choose lean fish and shellfish. But if you do not, go for oily fish, which are very healthy.

MONK-FISH CURRY

Prep time: 15 minutes
Cooking time: 20 minutes
Setting: Stew.
Serves: 2

Nutrition per serving:

Calories: 270	Sugar: 6	Protein: 45
Carbs: 16	Fat: 11	GL: 12

Ingredients:
- 0.5lb monk-fish
- 1 thinly sliced sweet yellow onion
- 0.5 cup chopped tomato
- 3tbsp strong curry paste
- 1tbsp oil or ghee

Recipe:
1. Set the Instant Pot to saute and add the onion, oil, and curry paste.
2. When the onion is soft, add the remaining ingredients and seal.
3. Cook on Stew for 20 minutes.
4. Release the pressure naturally.

SALMON BAKE

Prep time: 15 minutes
Cooking time: 15 minutes
Setting: Steam
Serves: 2

Nutrition per serving:

Calories: 260	Sugar: 1	Protein: 36
Carbs: 5	Fat: 12	GL: 1

Ingredients:

- 1lb salmon
- 1lb chopped Mediterranean vegetables
- 1 cup low sodium fish broth
- juice of half a lemon
- sea salt as desired

Recipe:
1. Mix all the ingredients except the broth in a foil pouch.
2. Place the pouch in the steamer basket your Instant Pot.
3. Pour the broth into your Instant Pot.
4. Cook on Steam for 15 minutes.
5. Release the pressure naturally.

MIXED CHOWDER

Prep time: 15 minutes
Cooking time: 35 minutes
Nutrition per serving:

Setting: Stew
Serves: 2

| Calories: 320 | Sugar: 2 | Protein: 41 |
| Carbs: 9 | Fat: 16 | GL: 4 |

Ingredients:
- 1lb fish stew mix
- 2 cups white sauce
- 3tbsp old bay seasoning

Recipe:
1. Mix all the ingredients in your Instant Pot.
2. Cook on Stew for 35 minutes.
3. Release the pressure naturally.

TROUT BAKE

Prep time: 15 minutes
Cooking time: 35 minutes
Nutrition per serving:

Setting: Steam
Serves: 2

| Calories: 310 | Sugar: 2 | Protein: 40 |
| Carbs: 14 | Fat: 12 | GL: 5 |

Ingredients:

- 1lb trout fillets, boneless
- 1lb chopped winter vegetables
- 1 cup low sodium fish broth
- 1tbsp mixed herbs
- sea salt as desired

Recipe:
1. Mix all the ingredients except the broth in a foil pouch.
2. Place the pouch in the steamer basket your Instant Pot.
3. Pour the broth into the Instant Pot.
4. Cook on Steam for 35 minutes.
5. Release the pressure naturally.

TUNA SWEETCORN CASSEROLE

Prep time: 15 minutes
Cooking time: 35 minutes
Setting: Stew
Serves: 2

Nutrition per serving:

Calories: 300   Sugar: 1   Protein: 43
Carbs: 6   Fat: 9   GL: 2

Ingredients:
- 3 small tins of tuna
- 0.5lb sweetcorn kernels
- 1lb chopped vegetables
- 1 cup low sodium vegetable broth
- 2tbsp spicy seasoning

Recipe:
1. Mix all the ingredients in your Instant Pot.
2. Cook on Stew for 35 minutes.
3. Release the pressure naturally.

SWORDFISH STEAK

Prep time: 15 minutes
Cooking time: 35 minutes
Setting: Steam
Serves: 2

Nutrition per serving:

Calories: 270   Sugar: 1   Protein: 48
Carbs: 5   Fat: 10   GL: 1

Ingredients:
- 1lb swordfish steak, whole
- 1lb chopped Mediterranean vegetables
- 1 cup low sodium fish broth
- 2tbsp soy sauce

Recipe:
1. Mix all the ingredients except the broth in a foil pouch.
2. Place the pouch in the steamer basket for your Instant Pot.
3. Pour the broth into the Instant Pot. Lower the steamer basket into the Instant Pot.
4. Cook on Steam for 35 minutes.
5. Release the pressure naturally.

SHRIMP COCONUT CURRY

Prep time: 15 minutes
Cooking time: 20 minutes
Setting: Stew.
Serves: 2

Nutrition per serving:

Calories: 380	Sugar: 4	Protein: 40
Carbs: 13	Fat: 22	GL: 14

Ingredients:
- 0.5lb cooked shrimp
- 1 thinly sliced onion
- 1 cup coconut yogurt
- 3tbsp curry paste
- 1tbsp oil or ghee

Recipe:
1. Set the Instant Pot to saute and add the onion, oil, and curry paste.
2. When the onion is soft, add the remaining ingredients and seal.
3. Cook on Stew for 20 minutes.
4. Release the pressure naturally.

TUNA AND CHEDDAR

Prep time: 15 minutes
Cooking time: 35 minutes
Setting: Stew
Serves: 2

Nutrition per serving:

Calories: 320	Sugar: 2	Protein: 37
Carbs: 8	Fat: 11	GL: 4

Ingredients:

- 3 small cans tuna
- 1lb finely chopped vegetables
- 1 cup low sodium vegetable broth
- 0.5 cup shredded cheddar

Recipe:

1. Mix all the ingredients in your Instant Pot.
2. Cook on Stew for 35 minutes.
3. Release the pressure naturally.

CHILI SHRIMP

Prep time: 15 minutes

Cooking time: 35 minutes

Setting: Stew

Serves: 2

Nutrition per serving:

Calories: 270	Sugar: 4	Protein: 51
Carbs: 6	Fat: 8	GL: 2

Ingredients:

- 1.5lb cooked shrimp
- 1lb stir fry vegetables
- 1 cup ready-mixed fish sauce
- 2tbsp chili flakes

Recipe:

1. Mix all the ingredients in your Instant Pot.
2. Cook on Stew for 35 minutes.
3. Release the pressure naturally.

SARDINE CURRY

Prep time: 15 minutes

Cooking time: 35 minutes

Setting: Stew

Serves: 2

Nutrition per serving:

Calories: 320	Sugar: 2	Protein: 42
Carbs: 8	Fat: 16	GL: 3

Ingredients:

- 5 tins of sardines in tomato
- 1lb chopped vegetables
- 1 cup low sodium fish broth
- 3tbsp curry paste

Recipe:

1. Mix all the ingredients in your Instant Pot.
2. Cook on Stew for 35 minutes.
3. Release the pressure naturally.

MUSSELS AND SPAGHETTI SQUASH

Prep time: 15 minutes   **Setting:** Stew
Cooking time: 35 minutes   **Serves:** 2

Nutrition per serving:

Calories: 265	Sugar: 1	Protein: 48
Carbs: 7	Fat: 9	GL: 3

Ingredients:

- 1lb cooked, shelled mussels
- 1/2 a spaghetti squash, to fit the Instant Pot
- 1 cup low sodium fish broth
- 3tbsp crushed garlic
- sea salt to taste

Recipe:

1. Mix the mussels with the garlic and salt.
2. Place the mussels inside the squash.
3. Lower the squash into your Instant Pot.
4. Pour the broth around it.
5. Cook on Stew for 35 minutes.
6. Release the pressure naturally.
7. Shred the squash, mixing the "spaghetti" with the mussels.

COD IN WHITE SAUCE

Prep time: 15 minutes
Cooking time: 5 minutes

Setting: Stew
Serves: 2

Nutrition per serving:

Calories: 390

Sugar: 2

Protein: 41

Carbs: 10

Fat: 26

GL: 5

Ingredients:
- 1lb cod fillets
- 1lb chopped swede and carrots
- 2 cups white sauce
- 1 cup peas
- 3tbsp black pepper

Recipe:
1. Mix all the ingredients in your Instant Pot.
2. Cook on Stew for 5 minutes.
3. Release the pressure naturally.

LEMON SOLE

Prep time: 15 minutes
Cooking time: 5 minutes

Setting: Stew
Serves: 2

Nutrition per serving:

Calories: 230

Sugar: 1

Protein: 46

Carbs: 4

Fat: 6

GL: 1

Ingredients:
- 1lb sole fillets, boned and skinned
- 1 cup low sodium fish broth
- 2 shredded sweet onions
- juice of half a lemon
- 2tbsp dried cilantro

Recipe:
1. Mix all the ingredients in your Instant Pot.
2. Cook on Stew for 5 minutes.
3. Release the pressure naturally.

COD IN PARSLEY SAUCE

Prep time: 15 minutes

Cooking time: 5 minutes

Setting: Stew

Serves: 2

Nutrition per serving:

Calories: 330
Sugar: 1
Protein: 40

Carbs: 8
Fat: 19
GL: 3

Ingredients:

- 1lb boneless, skinless cod fillets
- 0.5lb green peas
- 1 cup white sauce
- juice of a lemon
- 2tbsp dry parsley

Recipe:

1. Mix all the ingredients in your Instant Pot.
2. Cook on Stew for 35 minutes.
3. Release the pressure naturally.

CRAB CURRY

Prep time: 15 minutes

Cooking time: 20 minutes

Setting: Stew.

Serves: 2

Nutrition per serving:

Calories: 250
Sugar: 4
Protein: 24

Carbs: 11
Fat: 10
GL: 9

Ingredients:

- 0.5lb chopped crab
- 1 thinly sliced red onion
- 0.5 cup chopped tomato
- 3tbsp curry paste
- 1tbsp oil or ghee

Recipe:

1. Set the Instant Pot to saute and add the onion, oil, and curry paste.
2. When the onion is soft, add the remaining ingredients and seal.
3. Cook on Stew for 20 minutes.
4. Release the pressure naturally.

Vegetable Dishes

Whether you're a vegetarian, a vegan, or just plain sick and tired of eating meat and two veg for every single meal, you've probably wondered whether you can juggle your low carb needs whilst eating a plant based diet. It is definitely possible, but it's all about balance and about avoiding filling your plate with grains.

SQUASH MEDLEY

Prep time: 10 minutes.
Cooking time: 20 minutes.
Setting: Saute.
Serves: 2
Nutrition per serving:

Calories: 100	Sugar: 3	Protein: 5
Carbs: 10	Fat: 6	GL: 20

Ingredients:
- 2lbs mixed squash
- 0.5 cup mixed veg
- 1 cup vegetable stock
- 2tbsp olive oil
- 2tbsp mixed herbs

Recipe:
1. Put the squash in the steamer basket and add the stock into the Instant Pot.
2. Steam the squash in your Instant Pot for 10 minutes.
3. Depressurize and pour away the remaining stock.
4. Set to saute and add the oil and remaining ingredients.
5. Cook until a light crust forms.

EGGPLANT CURRY

Prep time: 15 minutes
Cooking time: 20 minutes
Setting: Stew.
Serves: 2
Nutrition per serving:

Calories: 350	Fat: 25
Carbs: 15	Protein: 11
Sugar: 3	GL: 10

Ingredients:
- 2-3 cups chopped eggplant
- 1 thinly sliced onion
- 1 cup coconut milk
- 3tbsp curry paste
- 1tbsp oil or ghee

Recipe:
1. Set the Instant Pot to saute and add the onion, oil, and curry paste.
2. When the onion is soft, add the remaining ingredients and seal.
3. Cook on Stew for 20 minutes. Release the pressure naturally.

CHICKPEA SOUP

Prep time: 15 minutes
Cooking time: 35 minutes
Nutrition per serving:

Setting: Stew
Serves: 2

Calories: 310	Sugar: 3	Protein: 27
Carbs: 20	Fat: 5	GL: 5

Ingredients:
- 1lb cooked chickpeas
- 1lb chopped vegetables
- 1 cup low sodium vegetable broth
- 2tbsp mixed herbs

Recipe:
1. Mix all the ingredients in your Instant Pot.
2. Cook on Stew for 35 minutes.
3. Release the pressure naturally.

FRIED TOFU HOTPOT

Prep time: 15 minutes
Cooking time: 15 minutes
Nutrition per serving:

Setting: Stew
Serves: 2

Calories: 320	Sugar: 3	Protein: 47
Carbs: 11	Fat: 23	GL: 6

Ingredients:

- 0.5lb fried tofu
- 1lb chopped Chinese vegetable mix
- 1 cup low sodium vegetable broth
- 2tbsp 5 spice seasoning
- 1tbsp smoked paprika

Recipe:
1. Mix all the ingredients in your Instant Pot.
2. Cook on Stew for 15 minutes.
3. Release the pressure naturally.

PEA AND MINT SOUP

Prep time: 15 minutes
Cooking time: 35 minutes
Setting: Stew
Serves: 2
Nutrition per serving:

| Calories: 130 | Sugar: 4 | Protein: 19 |
| Carbs: 17 | Fat: 5 | GL: 11 |

Ingredients:
- 1lb green peas
- 2 cups low sodium vegetable broth
- 3tbsp mint sauce

Recipe:
1. Mix all the ingredients in your Instant Pot.
2. Cook on Stew for 35 minutes.
3. Release the pressure naturally.
4. Blend into a rough soup.

LENTIL AND EGGPLANT STEW

Prep time: 15 minutes
Cooking time: 35 minutes
Setting: Stew
Serves: 2
Nutrition per serving:

| Calories: 310 | Sugar: 6 | Protein: 32 |
| Carbs: 22 | Fat: 10 | GL: 16 |

Ingredients:
- 1lb eggplant
- 1lb dry lentils
- 1 cup chopped vegetables
- 1 cup low sodium vegetable broth

Recipe:
1. Mix all the ingredients in your Instant Pot.
2. Cook on Stew for 35 minutes.
3. Release the pressure naturally.

TOFU CURRY

Prep time: 15 minutes
Cooking time: 20 minutes
Setting: Stew.
Serves: 2

Nutrition per serving:

| Calories: 300 | Sugar: 4 | Protein: 42 |
| Carbs: 9 | Fat: 14 | GL: 7 |

Ingredients:
- 2 cups cubed extra firm tofu
- 2 cups mixed stir fry vegetables
- 0.5 cup soy yogurt
- 3tbsp curry paste
- 1tbsp oil or ghee

Recipe:
1. Set the Instant Pot to saute and add the oil and curry paste.
2. When the onion is soft, add the remaining ingredients except the yogurt and seal.
3. Cook on Stew for 20 minutes.
4. Release the pressure naturally and serve with a scoop of soy yogurt.

FAKE-ON STEW

Prep time: 15 minutes
Cooking time: 25 minutes
Setting: Stew
Serves: 2

Nutrition per serving:

| Calories: 200 | Carbs: 12 | Sugar: 3 |

Fat: 7   Protein: 41   GL: 5

Ingredients:
- 0.5lb soy bacon
- 1lb chopped vegetables
- 1 cup low sodium vegetable broth
- 1tbsp nutritional yeast

Recipe:
1. Mix all the ingredients in your Instant Pot.
2. Cook on Stew for 25 minutes.
3. Release the pressure naturally.

LENTIL AND CHICKPEA CURRY

Prep time: 15 minutes
Cooking time: 20 minutes
Nutrition per serving:

Setting: Stew.
Serves: 2

Calories: 360	Sugar: 6	Protein: 23
Carbs: 26	Fat: 19	GL: 10

Ingredients:
- 2 cups dry lentils and chickpeas
- 1 thinly sliced onion
- 1 cup chopped tomato
- 3tbsp curry paste
- 1tbsp oil or ghee

Recipe:
1. Set the Instant Pot to saute and add the onion, oil, and curry paste.
2. When the onion is soft, add the remaining ingredients and seal.
3. Cook on Stew for 20 minutes.
4. Release the pressure naturally.

SEITAN ROAST

Prep time: 15 minutes
Cooking time: 35 minutes
Nutrition per serving:

Setting: Stew
Serves: 2

Calories: 260   Carbs: 9   Sugar: 2

Fat: 2   Protein: 49   GL: 4

Ingredients:

- 1lb seitan roulade
- 1lb chopped winter vegetables
- 1 cup low sodium vegetable broth
- 4tbsp roast rub

Recipe:

1. Rub the roast rub into your roulade.
2. Place the roulade and vegetables in your Instant Pot.
3. Add the broth. Seal.
4. Cook on Stew for 35 minutes.
5. Release the pressure naturally.

CHILI SIN CARNE

Prep time: 15 minutes
Cooking time: 35 minutes
Setting: Beans
Serves: 2
Nutrition per serving:

Calories: 240   Sugar: 5   Protein: 36
Carbs: 20   Fat: 3   GL: 11

Ingredients:

- 3 cups mixed cooked beans
- 2 cups chopped tomatoes
- 1tbsp yeast extract
- 2 squares very dark chocolate
- 1tbsp red chili flakes

Recipe:

1. Mix all the ingredients in your Instant Pot.
2. Cook on Beans for 35 minutes.
3. Release the pressure naturally.

MEATLESS BALL SOUP

Prep time: 15 minutes
Cooking time: 15 minutes
Setting: Stew
Serves: 2

Nutrition per serving:

Calories: 240
Carbs: 9

Sugar: 3
Fat: 10

Protein: 35
GL: 5

Ingredients:
- 1lb minced tofu
- 0.5lb chopped vegetables
- 2 cups low sodium vegetable broth
- 1tbsp almond flour
- salt and pepper

Recipe:
1. Mix the tofu, flour, salt and pepper.
2. Form the meatballs.
3. Place all the ingredients in your Instant Pot.
4. Cook on Stew for 15 minutes.
5. Release the pressure naturally.

SEITAN CURRY

Prep time: 15 minutes
Cooking time: 20 minutes

Setting: Stew.
Serves: 2

Nutrition per serving:

Calories: 240
Carbs: 19

Sugar: 4
Fat: 10

Protein: 32
GL: 10

Ingredients:
- 0.5lb seitan
- 1 thinly sliced onion
- 1 cup chopped tomato
- 3tbsp curry paste
- 1tbsp oil or ghee

Recipe:
1. Set the Instant Pot to saute and add the onion, oil, and curry paste.
2. When the onion is soft, add the remaining ingredients and seal.
3. Cook on Stew for 20 minutes.
4. Release the pressure naturally.

SPLIT PEA STEW

Prep time: 5 minutes   **Setting:** Beans
Cooking time: 35 minutes   **Serves:** 2
Nutrition per serving:

Calories: 300	Sugar: 3	Protein: 24
Carbs: 7	Fat: 2	GL: 4

Ingredients:
- 1 cup dry split peas
- 1lb chopped vegetables
- 1 cup mushroom soup
- 2tbsp old bay seasoning

Recipe:
1. Mix all the ingredients in your Instant Pot.
2. Cook on Beans for 35 minutes.
3. Release the pressure naturally.

MANGO TOFU CURRY

Prep time: 15 minutes   **Setting:** Stew
Cooking time: 35 minutes   **Serves:** 2
Nutrition per serving:

Calories: 310	Sugar: 9	Protein: 37
Carbs: 20	Fat: 4	GL: 19

Ingredients:
- 1lb cubed extra firm tofu
- 1lb chopped vegetables
- 1 cup low carb mango sauce
- 1 cup vegetable broth
- 2tbsp curry paste

Recipe:
1. Mix all the ingredients in your Instant Pot.
2. Cook on Stew for 35 minutes.
3. Release the pressure naturally.

Soups, Broths & Stews

Soups, broths, and stews are a great way of having extra fluid and minerals. The stock provides plenty of rich sauce and the vegetables and proteins, cooked down to perfection, provide much needed vitamins, minerals, and protein. All this helps you to focus on a lower carb, lower fat meal full of flavor and nutritional value. Besides this, creating a stew in your Instant Pot is super simple.

CHILI CON CARNE

Prep time: 15 minutes
Cooking time: 35 minutes
Nutrition per serving:

Setting: Stew
Serves: 2

Calories: 340   Sugar: 6   Protein: 46
Carbs: 16   Fat: 12   GL: 14

Ingredients:
- 1lb minced beef
- 1 cup mixed beans
- 2 cups chopped tomatoes
- 3 squares very dark chocolate
- 3tbsp mixed seasoning

Recipe:
1. Mix all the ingredients in your Instant Pot.
2. Cook on Stew for 35 minutes.
3. Release the pressure naturally.
4.

KIDNEY BEAN STEW

Prep time: 15 minutes
Cooking time: 15 minutes
Nutrition per serving:

Setting: Stew
Serves: 2

Calories: 270   Sugar: 3   Protein: 23
Carbs: 16   Fat: 10   GL: 8

Ingredients:
- 1lb cooked kidney beans
- 1 cup tomato passata
- 1 cup low sodium beef broth

- 3tbsp Italian herbs

Recipe:
1. Mix all the ingredients in your Instant Pot.
2. Cook on Stew for 15 minutes.
3. Release the pressure naturally.

CABBAGE SOUP

Prep time: 15 minutes   **Setting:** Stew
Cooking time: 35 minutes   **Serves:** 2
Nutrition per serving:

Calories: 60	Sugar: 0	Protein: 4
Carbs: 2	Fat: 2	GL: 1

Ingredients:
- 1lb shredded cabbage
- 1 cup low sodium vegetable broth
- 1 shredded onion
- 2tbsp mixed herbs
- 1tbsp black pepper

Recipe:
1. Mix all the ingredients in your Instant Pot.
2. Cook on Stew for 35 minutes.
3. Release the pressure naturally.

PUMPKIN SPICE SOUP

Prep time: 10 minutes   **Setting:** Stew
Cooking time: 35 minutes   **Serves:** 2
Nutrition per serving:

Calories: 100	Sugar: 1	Protein: 3
Carbs: 7	Fat: 2	GL: 1

Ingredients:
- 1lb cubed pumpkin
- 1 cup low sodium vegetable broth
- 2tbsp mixed spice

Recipe:
1. Mix all the ingredients in your Instant Pot.
2. Cook on Stew for 35 minutes.
3. Release the pressure naturally.
4. Blend the soup.

CREAM OF TOMATO SOUP

Prep time: 15 minutes
Cooking time: 15 minutes

Setting: Stew
Serves: 2

Nutrition per serving:

Calories: 20
Carbs: 2
Sugar: 1

Fat: 0
Protein: 3
GL: 1

Ingredients:
- 1lb fresh tomatoes, chopped
- 1.5 cups low sodium tomato puree
- 1tbsp black pepper

Recipe:
1. Mix all the ingredients in your Instant Pot.
2. Cook on Stew for 15 minutes.
3. Release the pressure naturally.
4. Blend.

SHIITAKE SOUP

Prep time: 15 minutes
Cooking time: 35 minutes

Setting: Stew
Serves: 2

Nutrition per serving:

Calories: 70
Carbs: 5

Sugar: 1
Fat: 2

Protein: 2
GL: 1

Ingredients:
- 1 cup shiitake mushrooms
- 1 cup diced vegetables

- 1 cup low sodium vegetable broth
- 2tbsp 5 spice seasoning

Recipe:
1. Mix all the ingredients in your Instant Pot.
2. Cook on Stew for 35 minutes.
3. Release the pressure naturally.

SPICY PEPPER SOUP

Prep time: 15 minutes
Cooking time: 15 minutes
Setting: Stew
Serves: 2
Nutrition per serving:

Calories: 100	Sugar: 4	Protein: 3
Carbs: 11	Fat: 2	GL: 6

Ingredients:
- 1lb chopped mixed sweet peppers
- 1 cup low sodium vegetable broth
- 3tbsp chopped chili peppers
- 1tbsp black pepper

Recipe:
1. Mix all the ingredients in your Instant Pot.
2. Cook on Stew for 15 minutes.
3. Release the pressure naturally. Blend.

ZOODLE WON-TON SOUP

Prep time: 15 minutes
Cooking time: 5 minutes
Setting: Stew
Serves: 2
Nutrition per serving:

Calories: 300	Sugar: 1	Protein: 43
Carbs: 6	Fat: 9	GL: 2

Ingredients:

- 1lb spiralized zucchini
- 1 pack unfried won-tons
- 1 cup low sodium beef broth
- 2tbsp soy sauce

Recipe:
1. Mix all the ingredients in your Instant Pot.
2. Cook on Stew for 5 minutes.
3. Release the pressure naturally.

BROCCOLI STILTON SOUP

Prep time: 15 minutes
Cooking time: 35 minutes
Nutrition per serving:

Setting: Stew
Serves: 2

Calories: 280
Carbs: 9

Sugar: 2
Fat: 22

Protein: 13
GL: 4

Ingredients:
- 1lb chopped broccoli
- 0.5lb chopped vegetables
- 1 cup low sodium vegetable broth
- 1 cup Stilton

Recipe:
1. Mix all the ingredients in your Instant Pot.
2. Cook on Stew for 35 minutes.
3. Release the pressure naturally.
4. Blend the soup.

LAMB STEW

Prep time: 15 minutes
Cooking time: 35 minutes
Nutrition per serving:

Setting: Stew
Serves: 2

Calories: 320
Carbs: 10

Sugar: 2
Fat: 8

Protein: 42
GL: 3

Ingredients:
- 1lb diced lamb shoulder

- 1lb chopped winter vegetables
- 1 cup low sodium vegetable broth
- 1tbsp yeast extract
- 1tbsp star anise spice mix

Recipe:
1. Mix all the ingredients in your Instant Pot.
2. Cook on Stew for 35 minutes.
3. Release the pressure naturally.

IRISH STEW

Prep time: 15 minutes
Cooking time: 35 minutes
Setting: Stew
Serves: 2
Nutrition per serving:

Calories: 330	Sugar: 2	Protein: 49
Carbs: 9	Fat: 12	GL: 3

Ingredients:
- 1.5lb diced lamb shoulder
- 1lb chopped vegetables
- 1 cup low sodium beef broth
- 3 minced onions
- 1tbsp ghee

Recipe:
1. Mix all the ingredients in your Instant Pot.
2. Cook on Stew for 35 minutes.
3. Release the pressure naturally.

SWEET AND SOUR SOUP

Prep time: 15 minutes
Cooking time: 35 minutes
Setting: Stew
Serves: 2
Nutrition per serving:

Calories: 270	Sugar: 9	Protein: 36
Carbs: 22	Fat: 2	GL: 12

Ingredients:
- 1lb cubed chicken breast
- 1lb chopped vegetables
- 1 cup low carb sweet and sour sauce
- 0.5 cup diabetic marmalade

Recipe:
1. Mix all the ingredients in your Instant Pot.
2. Cook on Stew for 35 minutes.
3. Release the pressure naturally.

MEATBALL STEW

Prep time: 15 minutes
Cooking time: 25 minutes
Setting: Stew
Serves: 2

Nutrition per serving:

Calories: 300	Sugar: 1	Protein: 40
Carbs: 4	Fat: 12	GL: 2

Ingredients:
- 1lb sausage meat
- 2 cups chopped tomato
- 1 cup chopped vegetables
- 2tbsp Italian seasonings
- 1tbsp vegetable oil

Recipe:
1. Roll the sausage into meatballs.
2. Put the Instant Pot on Saute and fry the meatballs in the oil until brown.
3. Mix all the ingredients in your Instant Pot.
4. Cook on Stew for 25 minutes.
5. Release the pressure naturally.

KEBAB STEW

Prep time: 15 minutes
Cooking time: 35 minutes
Setting: Stew
Serves: 2

Nutrition per serving:

Calories: 290   Sugar: 4   Protein: 34
Carbs: 22   Fat: 10   GL: 6

Ingredients:

- 1lb cubed, seasoned kebab meat
- 1lb cooked chickpeas
- 1 cup low sodium vegetable broth
- 1tbsp black pepper

Recipe:

1. Mix all the ingredients in your Instant Pot.
2. Cook on Stew for 35 minutes.
3. Release the pressure naturally.

FRENCH ONION SOUP

Prep time: 35 minutes   **Setting:** Stew
Cooking time: 35 minutes   **Serves:** 2
Nutrition per serving:
Calories: 110   Sugar: 3   Protein: 3
Carbs: 8   Fat: 10   GL: 4

Ingredients:

- 6 onions, chopped finely
- 2 cups vegetable broth
- 2tbsp oil
- 2tbsp Gruyere

Recipe:

1. Place the oil in your Instant Pot and cook the onions on Saute until soft and brown.
2. Mix all the ingredients in your Instant Pot.
3. Cook on Stew for 35 minutes.
4. Release the pressure naturally.

Hypo Snacks

Going into hypoglycemia is an experience nobody relishes. When you are diabetic, whatever your type of diabetes, you are at risk of it. When you have Type 2 diabetes you are most at risk from taking too much insulin, and the easiest fix is to eat some sugar. In this chapter we have some healthy, carby snacks for you to raise your blood sugar.

SWEET POTATO FRIES

Prep time: 10 minutes
Cooking time: 15 minutes

Setting: Saute.
Serves: 2

Nutrition per serving:

Calories: 250   Sugar: 17   Protein: 5
Carbs: 36   Fat: 7   GL: 30

Ingredients:
- 1lb sweet potato, cut into chips.
- 2tbsp butter
- 1tbsp olive oil
- 1tbsp honey
- salt and pepper

Recipe:
1. Blanch the potatoes in hot water.
2. Melt the butter and olive oil in the Instant Pot.
3. Add the sweet potato and saute until crisp.
4. Stir in the honey, salt and pepper. Leave to rest.

SUGAR OATS CUP

Prep time: 10 minutes
Cooking time: 5 minutes

Setting: Manual
Serves: 2

Nutrition per serving:

Calories: 220   Carbs: 35   Sugar: 11

Fat: 4   Protein: 10   GL: 23

Ingredients:
- 0.5 cup instant oats
- 2 cups milk
- 4tbsp brown sugar
- 1tsp cinnamon

Recipe:
1. Pour the milk into your Instant Pot.
2. Add the oats, sugar, and cinnamon, stir well.
3. Seal and close the vent.
4. Choose Manual and set to cook 5 minutes.
5. Release the pressure naturally.

LEEK AND POTATO SOUP

Prep time: 15 minutes   **Setting:** Stew.
Cooking time: 25 minutes   **Serves:** 2
Nutrition per serving:
Calories: 220   Sugar: 3   Protein: 5
Carbs: 26   Fat: 16   GL: 5

Ingredients:
- 2 cups chopped white potatoes
- 2 chopped leeks
- 1 cups vegetable stock
- 1 cup black pepper sauce
- 1 cup chopped cilantro

Recipe:
1. Mix all the ingredients in your Instant Pot.
2. Cook on Stew for 25 minutes.
3. Depressurize naturally and blend.

STUFFED APPLES

Prep time: 10 minutes   **Setting:** Steam
Cooking time: 20 minutes   **Serves:** 2
Nutrition per serving:
Calories: 129   Sugar: 15   Protein: 1
Carbs: 31   Fat: 0   GL: 16

Ingredients:

- 2 medium cooking apples
- 2oz blackberries
- 2tbsp honey
- 1/2tsp cinnamon

Recipe:

1. Core the apples, leaving a little at the base for structure.
2. Mix the honey, cinnamon, and blackberries, and pack into the apples.
3. Place the apples in the steamer basket in your Instant Pot.
4. Pour a cup of water into your Instant Pot.
5. Seal and cook on Steam 20 minutes.
6. Depressurize naturally.

BREAD AND BUTTER PUDDING

Prep time: 20 minutes
Cooking time: 20 minutes
Setting: Steam
Serves: 2

Nutrition per serving:

Calories: 560
Carbs: 40
Sugar: 29
Fat: 40
Protein: 9
GL: 30

Ingredients:

- 1 cup single cream
- 1 large egg
- 2 slices stale bread
- 1tbsp brown sugar
- 1tsp salted butter

Recipe:

1. Whisk together the egg, cream, and sugar.
2. Butter the bread and layer it in a small heat-proof bowl.
3. Pour the egg mix over the bread. Pour a cup of water into the Instant Pot.
4. Place the bowl in the steamer basket and the basket in the Instant Pot.
5. Cook on Steam, low pressure, for 20 minutes.
6. Depressurize quickly and serve.

HONEY OAT BOOST

Prep time: 10 minutes   **Setting:** Manual
Cooking time: 5 minutes   **Serves:** 2
Nutrition per serving:

| Calories: 320 | Sugar: 16 | Protein: 8 |
| Carbs: 37 | Fat: 4 | GL: 27 |

Ingredients:
- 0.5 cup instant oats
- 2 cups milk
- 4tbsp honey
- 2tbsp very milk chocolate chips

Recipe:
1. Pour the milk into your Instant Pot.
2. Add the oats, chocolate, and 3tbsp honey, stir well.
3. Seal and close the vent.
4. Choose Manual and set to cook 5 minutes.
5. Release the pressure naturally.
6. Drizzle with more honey.

EVE'S PUDDING

Prep time: 30 minutes   **Setting:** Steam.
Cooking time: 20 minutes   **Serves:** 2
Nutrition per serving:

| Calories: 600 | Sugar: 50 | Protein: 9 |
| Carbs: 75 | Fat: 30 | GL: 45 |

Ingredients:
- 2 large apples, thinly sliced
- 1 egg
- 3tbsp plain butter
- 3tbsp self-raising flour
- 2tbsp brown sugar

Recipe:
1. Grease a heat-proof bowl with a pinch of the butter and layer the apple into it.
2. Whisk the remaining butter and sugar together until it's blended.

3. Add in the eggs, then carefully fold in the flour. Spread the batter over the apples.
4. Pour a cup of water into the Instant Pot.
5. Place the bowl in the steamer basket and the basket in the Instant Pot.
6. Cook on Steam, low pressure, for 20 minutes. Depressurize quickly and serve.

JUICY LUCY

Prep time: 20 minutes
Cooking time: 15 minutes
Setting: Steam
Serves: 2
Nutrition per serving:

Calories: 276
Carbs: 56

Sugar: 16
Fat: 6

Protein: 3
GL: 27

Ingredients:
- 2 medium pears, peeled, cored, and quartered
- 3oz fruits of the forest, fresh or frozen-defrosted
- 1 tbsp blueberry jam
- 1 tbsp cake crumbs
- 1 tbsp brown sugar

Recipe:
1. Mix the fruits with the sugar and jam. Add the pears and mix them.
2. Put into a heat-proof bowl that fits in your steamer basket in your Instant Pot.
3. Pour a cup of water into the Instant Pot.
4. Place the bowl in the steamer basket and the basket in the Instant Pot.
5. Cook on Steam, low pressure, for 15 minutes. Depressurize quickly.
6. Mix the crumbs and butter, sprinkle over the pudding and serve.

APPLE CAKE

Prep time: 20 minutes

Cooking time: 20 minutes

Setting: Steam

Serves: 2

Nutrition per serving:

Calories: 185   Sugar: 12   Protein: 5

Carbs: 22   Fat: 8   GL: 12

Ingredients:

- 1 large chopped cooking apple
- 1tbsp flour
- 1tbsp butter
- 1 egg
- 1tsp sugar

Recipe:

1. Mix the butter and sugar. Add the egg, then fold in the flour. Fold in the apple.
2. Lightly grease a heat-proof bowl and pour the batter into the bowl.
3. Pour a cup of water into the Instant Pot.
4. Place the bowl in the steamer basket and the basket in the Instant Pot.
5. Cook on Steam, low pressure, for 20 minutes. Depressurize quickly and serve.

RICE PUDDING

Prep time: 10 minutes   **Setting:** Manual

Cooking time: 10 minutes   **Serves:** 2

Nutrition per serving:

Calories: 320   Sugar: 15   Protein: 2

Carbs: 45   Fat: 1   GL: 24

Ingredients:

- 0.5 cup dry white rice
- 2 cups milk
- 4tbsp sugar
- 1tsp vanilla extract

Recipe:

1. Pour the milk into your Instant Pot.
2. Add the remaining ingredients, stir well.
3. Seal and close the vent.
4. Choose Manual and set to cook 10 minutes.
5. Release the pressure naturally.

Desserts

This chapter is the complete opposite of the last one. When you're diabetic sometimes all you want is a delicious, sweet dessert. But eating dessert is not always easy, as most are high in simple sugars as well as fats. The desserts here are much lower in carbs and only moderate in fats, to give you a sweet treat for very little guilt.

PUMPKIN OATMEAL

Prep time: 10 minutes
Cooking time: 5 minutes
Nutrition per serving:
Calories: 320
Carbs: 14

Sugar: 2
Fat: 2

Setting: Manual
Serves: 2

Protein: 3
GL: 5

Ingredients:
- 1/4 cup oats
- 1 cup milk
- 1 cup pumpkin puree
- 4tbsp sweetener
- 1tsp cinnamon

Recipe:
1. Pour the milk into your Instant Pot.
2. Add the remaining ingredients, stir well. Seal and close the vent.
3. Choose Manual and set to cook 5 minutes. Release the pressure naturally.

WHITE CHOCOLATE

Prep time: 2 minutes
Cooking time: 2 minutes
Nutrition per serving:
Calories: 105
Carbs: 3

Sugar: 1
Fat: 12

Setting: Stew
Serves: 2

Protein: 4
GL: 1

Ingredients:
- 4tbsp double cream
- 6tsp powdered sweetener
- 3tsp sugar-free white chocolate mix
- hot water or fat-free milk

Recipe:
1. Mix all the ingredients in your Instant Pot.
2. Seal and cook on Stew for 2 minutes.
3. Depressurize naturally. Stir well and serve.

HOT CHOCOLATE

Prep time: 2 minutes   **Setting:** Stew
Cooking time: 2 minutes   **Serves:** 2
Nutrition per serving:

Calories: 100	Sugar: 1	Protein: 4
Carbs: 3	Fat: 11	GL: 1

Ingredients:
- 4tbsp double cream
- 6tsp powdered sweetener
- 3tsp sugar-free cocoa
- 1/4tsp vanilla extract
- hot water or fat-free milk

Recipe:
1. Mix all the ingredients in your Instant Pot.
2. Seal and cook on Stew for 2 minutes.
3. Depressurize naturally.
4. Stir well and serve.

RICH WILD RICE PUDDING

Prep time: 10 minutes   **Setting:** Manual
Cooking time: 10 minutes   **Serves:** 2
Nutrition per serving:

Calories: 320	Sugar: 2	Protein: 3
Carbs: 14	Fat: 2	GL: 5

Ingredients:
- 1/4 cup dry wild rice
- 1 cup milk
- 6 squares 90% dark chocolate

- 4tbsp sweetener
- 1tsp mixed spice

Recipe:
1. Pour the milk into your Instant Pot.
2. Add the remaining ingredients, stir well.
3. Seal and close the vent.
4. Choose Manual and set to cook 10 minutes.
5. Release the pressure naturally.

PEANUT BUTTER COOKIES

Prep time: 10 minutes **Setting:** Steam
Cooking time: 5 minutes **Serves:** 2
Nutrition per serving:

Calories: 390	Sugar: 9	Protein: 10
Carbs: 20	Fat: 26	GL: 7

Ingredients:
- 1/3 cup peanut butter
- 1/3 cup dark chocolate chips
- 2tbsp powdered sweetener
- 1tbsp applesauce
- pinch of baking soda

Recipe:
1. Mix the sweetener, applesauce, and baking soda together.
2. Add in the peanut butter.
3. Fold in the chocolate chips.
4. Make cookies and lay them out on a heat-proof tray that fits into your Instant Pot steamer tray.
5. Pour a cup of water into the Instant Pot.
6. Place the tray in the steamer basket and the basket in the Instant Pot.
7. Cook on Steam, low pressure, for 20 minutes.
8. Depressurize quickly and serve.
9.

CHIA PUDDING WITH MANGO

Prep time: 10 minutes **Setting:** Manual
Cooking time: 10 minutes **Serves:** 2

Nutrition per serving:

Calories: 320   Sugar: 5   Protein: 8
Carbs: 12   Fat: 6   GL: 7

Ingredients:

- 1/4 cup chia seeds
- 1 cup orange juice
- 1 cup chopped mango
- 4tbsp sweetener

Recipe:

1. Pour the milk into your Instant Pot.
2. Add the remaining ingredients, stir well.
3. Seal and close the vent.
4. Choose Manual and set to cook 10 minutes.
5. Release the pressure naturally.

LOW CARB CUSTARD

Prep time: 5 minutes   **Setting:** Steam
Cooking time: 20 minutes   **Serves:** 2

Nutrition per serving:

Calories: 273   Sugar: 0   Protein: 9
Carbs: 1.5   Fat: 27   GL: 1

Ingredients:

- 2 eggs
- 2oz cream cheese
- 1.5tbsp powdered sweetener
- 1.5tsp caramel sauce
- 1 cup water

Recipe:

1. Blend the ingredients together.
2. Pour into a heat-proof bowl that fits into your Instant Pot.
3. Pour a cup of water into the Instant Pot.
4. Place the bowl in the steamer basket and the basket in the Instant Pot.
5. Cook on Steam, low pressure, for 20 minutes.
6. Depressurize quickly and serve.

CHIA VANILLA PUDDING

Prep time: 10 minutes

Cooking time: 10 minutes

Setting: Manual

Serves: 2

Nutrition per serving:

Calories: 320   Sugar: 6   Protein: 8

Carbs: 11   Fat: 6   GL: 7

Ingredients:

- 1/4 cup chia seeds
- 2 cups milk
- 4tbsp sweetener
- 1tsp vanilla extract

Recipe:

1. Pour the milk into your Instant Pot.
2. Add the remaining ingredients, stir well.
3. Seal and close the vent.
4. Choose Manual and set to cook 10 minutes.
5. Release the pressure naturally.

CHILI CHOCOLATE

Prep time: 2 minutes

Cooking time: 2 minutes

Setting: Stew

Serves: 2

Nutrition per serving:

Calories: 100   Sugar: 1   Protein: 4

Carbs: 3   Fat: 11   GL: 1

Ingredients:

- 4tbsp double cream
- 3tsp powdered sweetener
- 3tsp sugar-free pure cocoa
- 1/8tsp chili powder
- hot water or fat-free milk

Recipe:

1. Mix all the ingredients in your Instant Pot.
2. Seal and cook on Stew for 2 minutes.
3. Depressurize naturally.
4. Stir well and serve.

BRAN PORRIDGE

Prep time: 10 minutes

Cooking time: 10 minutes

Setting: Manual

Serves: 2

Nutrition per serving:

Calories: 320   Sugar: 4   Protein: 3

Carbs: 12   Fat: 2   GL: 4

Ingredients:

- 1/4 cup bran
- 1 cup milk
- 1 cup diabetic applesauce
- 4tbsp sweetener
- 1tsp cinnamon

Recipe:

1. Pour the milk into your Instant Pot.
2. Add the remaining ingredients, stir well.
3. Seal and close the vent.
4. Choose Manual and set to cook 10 minutes.
5. Release the pressure naturally.

Amazing 5-Ingredient Recipes As Bonus

CRAB LEGS IN THE INSTANT POT

Cooking Time: 5 Minutes　　　　　　　　**Yield: 4 Servings**

Ingredients

2.5 pounds of crab legs

2 cups of water

1 cup butter

¼ teaspoon of lemon juice +zest

4 garlic cloves, finely minced

Directions

1. In a small heatproof bowl, add butter, lemon zest, lemon juice, and garlic.
2. Place in microwave and melt it at high temperature. Set aside for further use.
3. Pour water in the instant pot. Set the trivet on top. Add legs to the instant pot.
4. Lock the lid of the instant Pot and seal the vent. Set timer for 3 minutes at high pressure.
5. Once the timer beeps, quick release the steam.
6. Take out the leg and then serve with butter garlic sauce. Enjoy.

BLUE CHEESE AND PEAR MELTS

Cooking Time: 2 Minutes　　　　　　　　**Yield: 2 Servings**

Ingredients

2 ounces cream cheese

1/4 cup kiwi, puree

2 small pears, thinly sliced

4 tablespoons blue cheese, crumbled

Directions

1. Place the ingredients in the instant pot. Lock the lid.
2. Set the timer to 1-2 minutes at high pressure. Release steam naturally. Stir and serve.

INSTANT POT GHEE

Cooking Time: 10 Minutes   **Yield: 4 Servings**

Ingredients

20 ounces unsalted butter

Directions

1. Turn on the sauté mode of the instant pot and add butter to the pot.
2. The butter will start to melt, and turn milky and frothy.
3. After 8 minutes, the froth will disappear, and then bubbles will form.
4. Turn off the instant pot at this stage. The cooking process will continue for about 2 minutes. The bottom of the pot should not look brownish if it does, then transfer the ghee to a bowl, and place it on a rack to cool down.
5. Strain the ghee, and then pour into a glass container for further use.

KETO INSTANT POT CHUNKY CHILI

Cooking Time: 30 Minutes   **Yield: 2 Servings**

Ingredients

2 pounds of beef, ground   1-1/2 cup beef broth
2 tablespoons of olive oil   1-1/2 cup canned dice tomatoes
4 garlic cloves, minced   1 cup zucchini squash, diced

Directions

1. Turn on the sauté mode of the instant pot. Pour olive oil to the pot and add ground beef.
2. Sauté it for 5 minutes.
3. Once beef is brown, add the garlic cloves, zucchini, and diced tomatoes.
4. Pour the broth and then lock the lid. Set timer for 25 minutes at high pressure.
5. Once timer beeps, release the steam naturally for 10 minutes. Stir and serve.

INSTANT POT INDIAN FISH CURRY

Cooking time: 5 minutes   **Yield: 4 servings**

Ingredients

4 tablespoons of coconut oil

8 teaspoons of curry powder

½ cup of green onion

1 cup of coconut milk

2 garlic cloves, minced

2 pounds of fish fillets, salmon

Directions

1. Turn on the sauté mode of the instant pot and pour coconut oil. Allow the oil to heat up.
2. Then add curry powder and garlic. Cook for a few seconds.
3. Next, add the fish and cook for 20 seconds. Add half of the coconut milk.
4. Lock the lid. Set timer for 3 minutes at high pressure.
5. Release the steam using the quick release and then open the pot.
6. Add in remaining coconut milk and turn on the sauté mode.
7. Cook for 3 minutes and serve with a garnish of green onions.

VANILLA AND PUMPKIN PUDDING

Cooking Time: 20 Minutes   **Yield: 2 Servings**

Ingredients

2 organic eggs

1/2 cup heavy whipping cream

3/4 cup stevia

16 ounces canned pumpkin puree

1 teaspoon vanilla extract

Directions

1. Grease a small steel pan with oil spray.
2. In a bowl, whisk eggs and then add stevia, cream, canned pumpkin puree, and vanilla extract. Transfer the mixture into the greased pan.
3. Place steaming rack or trivet in instant pot. Pour two cups of water in the instant pot
4. Adjust the pan on the rack.
5. Cover the pan and set the timer to 20 minutes at high pressure
6. Once timer beeps, quick release the steam. Open the instant pot lid.
7. Remove the foil and place steel pan on cooling rack. Chill for 6 hours before servings
8. Enjoy with additional whipping cream

GLUTEN-FREE ALMOND CAKE

Cooking Time: 40 Minutes   **Yield: 2 Servings**

Ingredients

1-1/2 cups of almond flour
1 teaspoon baking soda
1 teaspoon cinnamon

2 eggs, lightly whisked
1/3 cup coconut oil, melted
1/3 cup heavy whipping cream

Directions

1. Combine dry ingredient in a steel bowl and mix.
2. In another small heatproof bowl combine and whisk all the wet ingredients.
3. Combine ingredient of both the bowls. Pour two cups of water in the instant pot.
4. Place trivet in the instant pot. Adjust the batter bowl on top of the trivet.
5. Lock the lid and set the timer to 40 minutes at high pressure.
6. Release pressure naturally for 10 minutes, followed by a quick release
7. Let the cake cool and then serve.

PORK TENDERLOIN CHILI

Cooking Time: 45 Minutes   **Yield: 3 Servings**

Ingredients

1.5 pounds of pork tenderloin
14 ounces of beef broth
1 pound plum tomatoes, sliced

2 jalapeño chopped
1 tablespoon chili powder
Salt and pepper, to taste

Directions

1. Dump all the ingredients in the instant pot. Lock the lid of the pot. Set timer for 45 minutes at high pressure. Once timer beeps, release the steam naturally for 10 minutes.
2. Then quickly release the steam. Open the pot and then stir, serve.

BIG RED CHILI MIX

Cooking Time: 35 Minutes   **Yield: 4 Servings**

Ingredients

10 ounces of beef sirloin, ground

2 tablespoons of olive oil

35 ounces of crushed tomatoes, with liquid

1 red onion, chopped

1/4 teaspoon ground allspice

Salt and pepper, to taste

20 slices cheese, cheddar

Directions

1. Turn on sauté mode of instant pot and pour olive oil. Add beef and cook for 5 minutes.
2. Then add remaining ingredients. Lock the lid and set a timer to 30 minutes.
3. Once timer beeps, naturally release the steam. Open the pot and serve the stew.

YOGURT CHICKEN

Cooking Time: 20-25 Minutes

Yield: 1 Serving

Ingredients

¼ cup of Plain yogurt

¼ teaspoon of Garam Masala

¼ teaspoon of turmeric

1/3 teaspoon of garlic ginger paste

Salt and black pepper, to taste

1 pound of chicken breasts, boneless and skinless

Directions

1. In a bowl, mix all the ingredients and marinate the chicken for 40 minutes.
2. Pour two cups of water in the instant pot. Set the trivet inside the pot.
3. Cover the trivet bottom with aluminum foil.
4. Now place marinate chicken on a trivet above the foil.
5. Lock the lid of the pot and set the timer to 15 minutes at high pressure.
6. Once timer beeps, quick release the steam. Now transfer the chicken to the oil greased baking sheet. Broil the chicken in the oven at 375 degrees F until brown for 5-8 minutes.
7. Once done serve and enjoy.

BLUEBERRY-PEAR COMPOTE

Cooking Time: 8 Minutes   **Yield: 8 Servings**

Ingredients

6 pears, stem intact and peeled

2/3 cup stevia

1 lemon juice and zest

2 tablespoons butter

2 cups blueberries, thawed

Directions

1. Combine all the ingredients in the instant pot. Add ¼ cup of water. Stir ingredients well.
2. Cook on high pressure for 8 minutes. After timer beeps, quick release the steam.Serve.

POACHED PEACHES

Cooking Time: 4 Minutes   **Yield: 4 Servings**

Ingredients

4 cups of grapefruit juice

1 lemon, juice and zest

1 cinnamon stick

4 peaches, deseeded and peeled

Directions

1. Pour juice, cinnamon stick, water and lemon juice in the instant pot.
2. Peel the peaches and leave the stem intact. Cut in half and remove the seeds.
3. Now place the peaches in the instant pot.
4. Lock the lid and set the timer to 4 minutes at high pressure.
5. Then, naturally release the steam for 10 minutes, followed by quick release.
6. Open the pot and let the apricots get cooled down. Serve chilled.

WALNUTS AND RASPBERRIES BREAD

Cooking Time: 12 Minutes   **Yield: 4 Servings**

Ingredients

8 tablespoons of butter/coconut oil

1/3 teaspoon of cinnamon

1 cup walnuts, crushed

1 cup raspberries

1/3 cup of plain milk

2 cups of almond flour

Directions

1. Mix butter and cinnamon in a large mixing bowl.
2. Once fluffy, add walnuts, raspberries, milk, and almond flour.
3. Spoon the mixture to an oil greased small loaf pan. Pour two cups of water in the instant pot. Place trivet inside the pot. Place small loaf pan on top of the trivet.
4. Close the lid of the instant pot. Set timer for 8-12 minutes at high.
5. Once timer beeps, quick release the steam. Take out the pan.
6. Let the cake cool off. Then serve by slicing. Enjoy.

CHEESY SAUCE

Cooking Time: 7 Minutes   **Yield: 3 Servings**

Ingredients

¼ cup butter

Salt and black pepper, to taste

1/3 teaspoon onion powder

1 tablespoon tapioca starch

1 1/3 cups whole milk

2 cups sharp Cheddar cheese, grated

Directions

1. Turn on the sauté mode of the instant pot. Add butter and let it get warm.
2. Once the butter melts season it with salt and black pepper.
3. Then sprinkle tapioca starch and mix well.
4. Pour the milk gradually to the instant pot mixture and stir gently.
5. Once the ingredients reach the boiling temperature turns off the pot.
6. Turn on the keep warm setting and then add cheese and onion powder.
7. Let the cheese melt.
8. Once the ingredients are well blended, turn off the instant pot and serve the sauce.

BLUE CHEESE AND PEAR SPREAD

Cooking Time: 7 Minutes   **Yield: 2 Servings**

Ingredients

2 ounces cream cheese

2 tablespoons of butter

1/4 cup blueberry marmalade

1/2 small pear, thinly sliced

2 tablespoons crumbled blue cheese

¼ cup of milk, plain

Directions

1. Turn on the sauté mode of instant pot and add butter.
2. Then add cream cheese, blueberry marmalade, and blue cheese along with pears.
3. Sauté for 1 minute. Then add milk and keep on stirring until all the ingredients combined.
4. Turn on the keep warm and wait until it gets thick in texture. Then serve.

GOAT CHEESE AND SALAMI MELTS ON KETO BREAD

Cooking Time: 2 Minutes   **Yield: 2 Servings**

Ingredients

2 ounces goat cheese, reduced-fat

2–4 tablespoons sun-dried tomato pesto

2–3 ounces thinly sliced salami

2 slices of keto bread

Directions

1. Pour two cups of water in the instant pot. Adjust trivet inside the instant pot.
2. Take an aluminum foil and layer salami on it. Top the salami with pesto and goat cheese.
3. Wrap the foil around the salami and make a small pocket.
4. Place the aluminum foil on a trivet. Lock the lid of the instant pot. Set timer for 2 minutes at high. Once timer beeps, release the steam quickly and transfer foil to a plate.
5. The cheese melts till now. Open the foil. Place the mixture over the keto bread slices and serve. Enjoy.

INSTANT POT SALMON WITH JALAPENO

Cooking Time: 5 Minutes   **Yield: 2 Servings**

Ingredients

10 ounces of salmon fillet

Salt and black pepper, to taste

2 jalapeno seeds, minced

1 garlic clove

2 teaspoons of olive oil

1/2 teaspoon cumin

Directions

1. Combine salt, black pepper, jalapeno seeds, garlic cloves, olive oil and cumin in a bowl.
2. Pour 1-2 cups of water inside the instant pot. Set a steaming rack on top.
3. Cover the steaming rack with aluminum foil. Season the fillet with rub mixture.
4. Place the salmon on the steaming rack.
5. Lock the lid and set the timer to 5 minutes at high pressure.
6. Once the timer beeps, release the steam naturally.
7. Open the lid of the instant pot and then transfer the salmon to plate. Serve and enjoy.

KETO LOW CARB CHILI RECIPE

Cooking Time: 55 Minutes   **Yield: 6 Servings**

Ingredients

3 pounds of beef, ground

1 large onion

1 tablespoon of olive oil

4 cloves of garlic

2 can of tomatoes, diced

Salt and black pepper, to taste

1 cup beef bone broth, unsalted

Directions

1. Turn on the sauté mode of the instant pot and add oil and onions.
2. Cook the onions for 5 minutes until translucent. Then add garlic and cook for one minute.
3. Add ground beef and cook for 7 minutes. Then add remaining ingredients and stir.
4. Lock the lid of the instant pot. Set timer for 35 minutes at high pressure.
5. Once the timer beeps, release the steam naturally. Then quickly release the steam.
6. Once done serve.

HERBED TURKEY BREAST WITH BUTTER GRAVY

Cooking Time: 50 Minutes   **Yield: 2 Servings**

Ingredients

1.5 pounds of turkey breast   Salt & pepper
1 teaspoon of sage   1 cup of chicken broth
½ teaspoon of thyme   ½ cup of butter or oil
¼ teaspoon of dried rosemary

Directions

1. Mix sage, thyme, rosemary, salt and black pepper in a bowl.
2. Rub the turkey meat with the spices. Put the turkey breast in the instant pot.
3. Pour the broth in the instant pot and place lid on top of the instant pot.
4. Set the timer to high for 45 minutes.
5. Once timer beeps, release the steam naturally for 10 minutes.
6. Open the pot and take out the turkey, slice up the turkey breast.
7. Turn on sauté mode and evaporate gravy by adding butter. Serve with turkey.

KICKING CHICKEN

Cooking Time: 16minutes   **Yield: 2 Servings**

Ingredients

3 pounds of boneless, skinless   ½ cup medium salsa
chicken thighs   ¼ cup chopped fresh basil
¾ cup peanut butter,   1 tablespoon of almond flour
homemade

Directions

1. In a stainless steel bowl, combine chicken, peanut sauce, salsa, and basil.
2. Coat the chicken well. Place chicken in the instant pot and add 4 tablespoons of water.
3. Set nozzle to steaming position. Set timer for 12 minutes at high pressure.

4. Once timer beeps, quick release the steam. Remove chicken to a cutting board.
5. Let it cool. Turn on sauté mode of the instant pot and add almond flour.
6. Thick the sauce inside the pot.
7. Once it's, done, serve over cooked chicken.

The Final Words

When it comes to managing Type 2 diabetes it is incredibly important to make sure that you know yourself and your body first and foremost. A meal that is right for one person may not be right for another, and a food type you can eat for breakfast may not be as good at dinner time. For that reason, this book has included carb counts, sugar counts, and GL measures, to make sure that you are making an informed decision. When in doubt, stick to foods that are within your ideal range, which your doctor or nutritionist should be able to work out with you.

Likewise, if you have another type of diabetes your needs will be very different to someone with Type 2 diabetes. Some of the recipes in this book may not be right for you, as they may have too much fat, too many total carbs, or too many calories. If you have a different type of diabetes, again, discuss with your doctor or your nutritionist what nutritional balance your meals should have, and follow their guidelines, only eating meals that are right for you.

Hopefully this book has provided you with the tools you need to eat a safe, healthy diet as a Type 2 diabetic. As you can see, it is quick, simple, and delicious to eat a healthy diabetic diet, no matter what your tastes or needs are!

APPENDIX - MEASUREMENT CONVERSIONS

IMPERIAL	METRIC	CUPS
1oz	28g	8tsp
1lb	453.5	3.5 cups
1fl/oz	29.5ml	6tsp
1 gallon	3.8L	16 cups
0.03 oz	1 gram	0.25tsp
2.2lb	1 kilo	8 cups
0.3fl/oz	1 milliliter	0.2tsp
33.8fl/oz	1 liter	4.2 cups
1 inch	2.54cm	1tbsp
0.4 inch	1 cm	1tsp
0.17fl/oz	5ml	1tsp
0.5fl/oz	15ml	1tbsp
8fl/oz	236.5ml	1 cup

Made in the USA
Coppell, TX
20 September 2020